Atlas of Ear, Nose and Throat Diseases
including Bronchoesophagology
Second Edition

ATLAS OF EAR, NOSE AND THROAT DISEASES

INCLUDING BRONCHOESOPHAGOLOGY

WALTER BECKER, M.D.
Professor and Director of the University Clinic and Policlinic
for Ear, Nose and Throat Diseases, Bonn

RICHARD A. BUCKINGHAM, M.D.
Clinical Professor of Otolaryngology, Abraham Lincoln School of Medicine,
University of Illinois; Otologist, Resurrection Hospital, Chicago

PAUL H. HOLINGER, M.D.
Late Professor of Bronchoesophagology, Department of Otolaryngology,
Abraham Lincoln School of Medicine, University of Illinois, Chicago

WOLFGANG STEINER, M.D.
MICHAEL P. JAUMANN, M.D.
University Clinic for Ear, Nose and Throat Diseases, Erlangen

With a Contribution by
WALTER MESSERKLINGER, M.D.
Professor and Chief, University Ear, Nose and Throat Clinic, Graz

Edited by
WALTER BECKER, M.D.

Second Completely Revised Edition
With 866 Illustrations in Color, Partly Supplemented by 189 Drawings

1984
W. B. SAUNDERS COMPANY
Philadelphia ● Toronto ● Mexico City ● Rio de Janeiro ● Sydney

W. B. Saunders Company:

West Washington Square
Philadelphia, PA 19105

1 Goldthorne Avenue
Toronto, Ontario M8Z 5T9, Canada

Apartado 26370 – Cedro 512
Mexico 4, D. F., Mexico

Rua Coronel Cabrita, 8
Sao Cristovao Caixa Postal 21176
Rio de Janeiro, Brazil

9 Waltham Street
Artarmon, N.S.W. 2064, Australia

Original German edition: Atlas der Hals-Nasen-Ohren-Krankheiten
©1969, 1983 Georg Thieme Verlag, Stuttgart

Authorized English edition co-published by W. B. Saunders
Company, Philadelphia and Georg Thieme Verlag, Stuttgart

Important Note: Medicine is an ever-changing science. Research and clinical experience are continually broadening our knowledge, in particular our knowledge of proper treatment and drug therapy. Insofar as this book mentions any dosage or application, readers may rest assured that the authors, editors and publishers have made every effort to ensure that such references are strictly in accordance with the state of knowledge at the time of production of the book. Nevertheless, every user is requested to carefully examine the manufacturers' leaflets accompanying each drug to check on his own responsibility whether the dosage schedules recommended therein or the contraindications stated by the manufacturers differ from the statements made in the present book. Such examination is particularly important with drugs which are either rarely used or have been newly released on the market.

© 1969, 1984 Georg Thieme Verlag, P. O. Box 732, D-7000
Stuttgart 1, West Germany. Printed in Germany.

ISBN 3-13-576902-4 (Thieme)
ISBN 0-7216-1616-X (Saunders)
Library of Congress catalog card numer 82-80398

Preface to the Second English Edition

This is the second edition of this book, the first was published in six languages in 1969, and this edition in German and English in 1983.

Having worked with Professor Becker for five years on the first edition, I know firsthand, the careful and painstaking planning and editing that went into the first edition. Professor Becker began working on the second edition almost as soon as he had sent the final proofs to the Thieme Verlag in Stuttgart in 1969.

Becker's concept of an Atlas is that it should point out the salient, visual features of various disorders, assist the physician in recognition and understanding of these diseases and lead him to a correct diagnosis.

To produce an atlas that would not be out of date within a few years, he has eschewed references to therapies which are constantly being changed, improved and at times even eliminated. As he stressed in the Preface to the first edition, therapies may change radically but the need for correct, accurate diagnosis will always be constant. To this end, Becker has searched unceasingly and untiringly for the many new photographs he has gathered in this edition. His aim, which he expressed to me at the very start of this work, was to produce a book that would be as entirely new as possible.

As he noted in the Preface of this edition, fiberoptic endoscopic telescopes have been developed and perfected since the first edition was published, and he has included many examples obtained with these instruments in this book. Microscopic otoscopy has become the routine method of examining the pathologic ear within the period between the two editions, the otoscopic photographs taken with the Brubaker camera represent the findings as seen through the microscope even though the Brubaker camera does not use a microscope lens system.

I know from personal observation that Becker, with the eye of a highly experienced and expert art critic, has viewed, reviewed, selected and rejected literally thousands of color transparencies until he was satisfied that he had the best possible examples of otolaryngologic and head and neck diseases that could be seen by the aided and unaided eye.

He has insisted that the color reproductions be as perfect as the best artisans of the printing industry in Germany could make them.

Becker has spent much time agonizing over the order of presentation of the material. To him the logical sequence of the presentation of diseases in this book is almost as important, pedigogically, as the quality of the presentation.

The places of the late Professors P. H. HOLINGER and FRANCIS L. LEDERER, if indeed they could be replaced, have been taken by two young German Otolaryngologists, Priv. Doz. Dr. W. STEINER and Dr. M. P. JAUMANN, co-workers at the University Ear, Nose and Throat Clinic in Erlangen.

They have helped popularize and promulgate the use of the fiberoptic telescopes in the field of ear, nose and throat.

The contributions of Professor Dr. WALTER MESSER-KLINGER, Chairman of the University Ear, Nose and Throat Clinic, Graz, Austria merit special praise and thanks. A pioneer in the telescopic endoscopic study of the nose and paranasal sinuses, his excellent photographs have improved and modernized that section of this edition.

During these past almost twenty years, Professor BECKER has become my fast, respected and revered friend. I know he has devoted a large part of his professional life during this time to the perfection of this Atlas and am proud to have been associated with him in the endeavor.

Chicago, Fall, 1983

RICHARD A. BUCKINGHAM

Preface to the First English Edition

THERE IS ONLY ONE DIAGNOSIS BUT MANY FORMS OF THERAPY

The objective of this Atlas is embodied in this statement. It is accomplished through demonstration and documentation of otorhinolaryngologic and bronchoesophagologic pathology. Thus, the authors present a foundation upon which rational therapy may be developed. The major disease entities encountered in the specialty are depicted by suitable external photographs of the head and neck, as well as by endoscopic photographs of the tympanic membrane and middle ear, the epipharynx, larynx, and the lower air and food passages. In areas in which the use of the operating microscope has become standard practice, the camera has recorded the pathology with suitable magnification. Significant dermatologic conditions that have directly related as well as differential diagnostic importance are incorporated. In addition, radiology, including tomography, and histologic morphology are recognized as irreplaceable diagnostic components. However, it would have exceeded the scope of this Atlas if these two disciplines had been utilized to their fullest extent; yet in certain cases we have availed ourselves of these adjuvants as the need arose. Therapy is considered only in a few selected instances for better understanding of the progress of some of the disease states. An arbitrary arrangement of the material is maintained throughout each chapter, including identification of normal structures, congenital anomalies, neurogenic lesions, trauma, inflammatory diseases, and benign and malignant tumors.

The illustrations have been selected from photographic records accumulated during several decades of documenting clinical observations. Each picture is dependent on photographic equipment and technique, much of which was specially designed for the various types of illustrations. Full recognition to Joseph D. Brubaker, FBPA, and James E. Brubaker, FBPA, is hereby accorded for their pioneer work in developing and constructing endoscopic cameras used to obtain the color photographs of the ear, postnasal space, pharynx, larynx, tracheobronchial tree, and esophagus. This work was supported, in part, by The Jacques Holinger Memorial Fund.

In the Foreword to the German edition, the Editor, Professor Dr. Walter Becker, expresses his thanks to the coauthors; to an esteemed former chief, Professor Emeritus Dr. H. Leicher, Mainz; and to Professor Dr. A. Becker, Nürnberg; Professor Dr. H. G. Bönninghaus, Heidelberg; Professor Dr. F. Dallenbach, Heidelberg; Professor Dr. W. Doerr, Heidelberg; Professor Dr. O. Haferkamp, Bonn; Dozentin Dr. H. Hallerbach, Bonn; Professor Dr. H. H. Jansen, Heidelberg; and Professor Dr. P. Thurn, Bonn, all of whom have given their support and advice. L. T. Tenta, M.D., Assistant Professor of Otolaryngology, Chicago, and R. J. Blumenfeld, M.D., El Paso, Texas, contributed much to assembling and authenticating case histories. B. J. Soboroff, M.D.,

Professor of Otolaryngology, and W. L. Schmerold, M.D., Clinical Assistant in Dermatology, both of Chicago, gave valuable consultative help.

P. B. Szanto, M.D., whose particular interest has been otolaryngic pathology, gave valuable assistance in the identification, selction, and description of the histopathology. G. E. Valvassori, M.D., was responsible for the radiographs as well as the tomograms particularly significant to middleear and laryngeal pathology.

Maria E. Ikenberg, RBP, FBPA, Scientific Photographer at the Illinois Eye and Ear Infirmary, Department of Otolaryngology, University of Illinois, produced many of the illustrations of the pathology of the head and neck. We extend our thanks to her for aiding in the selection of material, for assistance in translations, and above all for the dedication to the innumerable tasks associated with the mechanics of setting up this Atlas. In addition, Christiane Heichen, Mainz, produced many of the photographs. Lotte Bär-Winnen, Bonn, gave invaluable help in various phases of the organization of this book as well as in translating. During its final stages Anneliese Karwel, Bonn, also aided. Elizabeth Lanzl, Park Forest, Illinois, provided important assistance in translation from the German text. Special mention and credit are extended to Karl H. Seeber, Tübingen, for the drawings which reflect his great ability and artistic understanding.

Credit for some of the illustrations is extended to D. F. Austin, M.D., Assistant Professor of Otolaryngology, Chicago; Professor Dr. J. L. Chamouard, Paris; Professor Dr. A. Ennuyer, Paris; S. A. Friedberg, M.D., Professor of Otolaryngology, Chicago; Professor Dr. C. H. Hamberger, Stockholm; Professor Dr. Dr. Kirstein, Stuttgart; P. C. Kronfeld, M.D., Professor of Ophthalmology, Chicago; Priv.-Doz. Dr. W. Maassen, Essen-Heidhausen; D. E. Ore, D.D.S., Assistant Professor of Pedodontics, Chicago; E. A. Petrus, M.D., Professor of Pathology, Chicago; S. Pruzansky, D.D.S., Professor of Dentistry, Chicago; Professor Dr. G. Seifert, Hamburg; Professor O. E. Van Alyea, M.D., Professor of Otolaryngology Emeritus, Chicago, and L. J. Wallner, M.D., Clinical Associate Professor of Otolaryngology, Chicago.

Special thanks go to Dr. med. h. c. Günther Hauff, of Georg Thieme Verlag, Stuttgart, who seven years ago encouraged the editor to undertake this project. Throughout the years he gave us the benefit of his friendship and vast publishing experience. The efficiency of his publishing house, as well as the assistance of his most able staff, especially Mr. G. Krüger, has helped made this book possible.

Appreciation is expressed to Mr. John L. Dusseau, Vice-President and Editor, W. B. Saunders Company, Philadelphia, for his cooperation in the preparation of this English edition.

WALTER BECKER, RICHARD A. BUCKINGHAM, PAUL H. HOLINGER, GÜNTER W. KORTING, FRANCIS L. LEDERER

Preface to the Second German Edition

"There are many forms of therapy, but only one diagnosis." The first edition of this Atlas, published in six languages, began with this sentence which still holds true today. Our aim in this second edition, as it was in the first, is to present the most comprehensive Atlas of Diseases of the Ear, Nose and Throat that we possibly can.

Development and improvement of the fiberoptic instruments and the operating microscope have greatly improved the visualization and diagnosis of diseases of the nose, paranasal sinuses, nasopharynx, larynx, and hypopharynx.

With these newer diagnostic instruments, blind spots in structures previously difficult to see have been to a great extent eliminated. Microlaryngoscopy, straight and flexible fiberoptic endoscopes have opened a new era in diagnosis and photographic documentation of diseases.

The illustrations in this book show the clinical and practical results obtained with these new instruments and techniques that the authors have helped develop.

What the physician sees with the head mirror is only the beginning of the ear, nose and throat examination, and today microscopic and telescopic examinations are almost an essential part of the complete ear, nose and throat examination.

We have continued the basic concept of the first edition to present subjects most important for the clinician. We have expanded the coverage of the different forms of secretory otitis and disturbances of middle ear aeration, since these disorders occur so frequently. Included in the chronic otitis media section is documentation of the formation of some types of cholesteatomas.

We have included examples of the frequently occurring complications of long term endotracheal intubation in the larynx and trachea. We have tried with many new illustrations to demonstrate the newest methods of early visualization and diagnosis of malignancies of the air and food passages which seem to be on the increase and continue to be seen by the physician in the advanced stages.

Roentgenology has been deemphasized, since the Thieme Verlag has just published the excellent book on Radiology of the Ear, Nose and Throat which complements this book. Some of the illustrations which we have taken from the first edition were reversed for technical reasons. We have tried to print only the best photographs possible. The quality of an illustration depends on many factors such as light source, film, exposure time, developing technique, the method of printing, offset in this edition, letter press in the first, and lighting conditions for the reader. For example note the difference in color reproduction in Figs. 87 and 88. We all understand that the reproduction of a photograph cannot perfectly represent the findings in the patient.

The tympanic membranes and many of the endoscopic photographs of the larynx, nasopharynx, bronchi and esophagus were taken with the camera developed by JOSEPH D. and JAMES E. BRUBAKER. Their contributions were noted in the Preface of the first edition.

The new telescopic photographs of the nasopharynx, pharynx, and larynx were taken with a reflex camera attached to the telescopes and designed by Stuckrad.

FRANCIS L. LEDERER, Chicago, died in 1973, and PAUL H. HOLINGER, Chicago, died in 1979. With their deaths we lost two of our authors of the first edition and Otolaryngology lost two outstanding teachers and clinicians. The continued use of some of their illustrations in this second edition is proof that the leadership of these two great men will live on. LAUREN D. HOLINGER, Chicago, continuing the work of his father, contributed Figures 670, 671, 680, 808, 809 and 815.

Many thanks to my coauthers whose clinical and photographic expertise made this edition possible.

The editorial work, intelligence and untiring assistance of Frau A. KARWEL was indispensible in the making of this book.

The following Doctors and Professors have contributed illustrations as indicated:
Dr. C. T. BUITER, Groningen, Figs. 397, 418; Dr. David W. BREWER, Chicago, Fig. 445; Prof. Dr. O. HORNSTEIN, Erlangen, Figs. 553, 560, 593, 594, 614, 620, 626, 628, 629, 630; Prof. Dr. H. JUNG, Koblenz, Figs. 59, 366, 475, 478, 496, 499, 709; Prof. Dr. KLINGMÜLLER, Bonn, Figs. 51, 310, 316, 318, 551, 563, 566, 586, 591, 597, 598, 601, 608, 615, 843; Prof. Dr. G. W. KORTING, Mainz, Figs. 25, 45, 47, 57, 60, 62, 63, 556, 568, 596, 621 and 31 Figs. of the first edition; Dr. E. LÖHLE and Dr. K. H. KOPP, Freiburg, Figs. 667, 668, 669; Dr. M. MINNEMANN, Bonn, Fig. 317; Prof. Dr. C. R. PFALTZ, Basel, Figs. 30, 363, 512, 529, 532, 754; Figs. 65 and 587 were taken by Frieboes, W. und W. SCHÖNFELD; Atlas der Haut- und Geschlechtskrankheiten, 3. Aufl., Thieme, Stuttgart, 1966.

Heartfelt thanks go to all of those mentioned above and especially to the Thieme Verlag, Stuttgart, to Herr Dr. med. h. c. G. HAUFF and to Herr G. KRÜGER.

Bonn, Fall, 1983   WALTER BECKER

Contents

Explanatory Note Concercing the Orientation of the Endoscopic Photographs in this Atlas

In the following schematic illustrations the findings in the nasopharynx and larynx are shown in the orientation that the physician sees during examinations with the mirror, in the eye piece of the rigid telescopes and in microscopic laryngoscopy.

To simplify the presentation of the nasopharynx and larynx, all such photographs have been oriented in a uniform manner. Thus the roof of the nasopharynx and anterior commissure of the larynx are rotated in all the illustrations so that they appear on the superior margin of the photographs.

The right angle telescopic views are therefore rotated 180° as demonstrated in Example II for the nasopharynx and Example V for the larynx.

When oriented in this manner with the microlaryngoscopic and the telescopic images of the larynx, the right side of the photograph shows the right side of the patient and vice versa.

With mirror views of the nasopharynx and larynx the right side of the photograph shows the left side of the patient and vice versa.

Nasopharynx

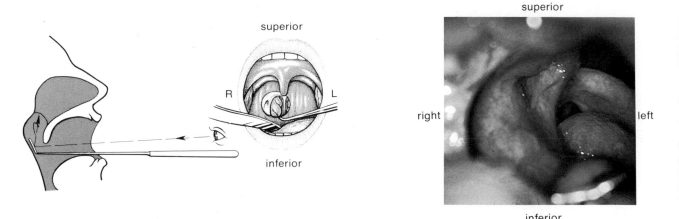

Example I: Mirror nasopharyngoscopy: Anatomy of the right eustachian tube orifice and choana.

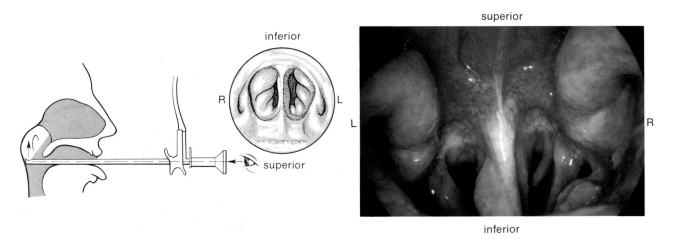

Example II: Telescopic nasopharyngoscopy: Normal nasopharynx

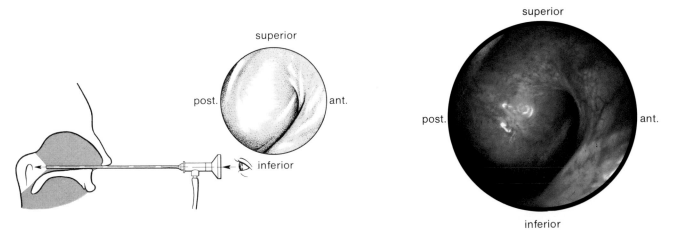

Example III: Telescopic view: Eustachian tube orifice at rest, left.

Larynx

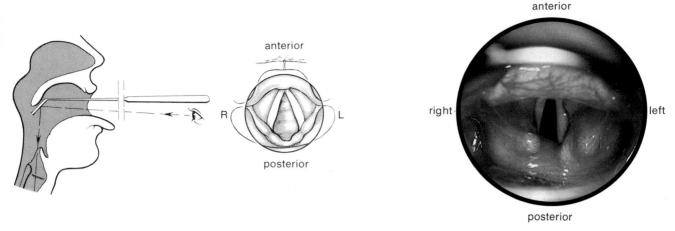

Example IV: Mirror laryngoscopy: View following right arytenoidectomy with lateral fixation of right vocal cord.

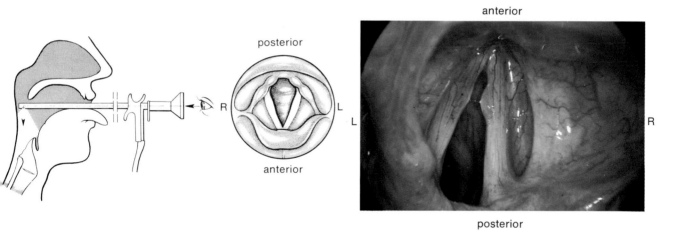

Example V: Telescopic laryngoscopy: View of right laryngeal ventricle and fine blood vessels of ventricle. There is also a singer's node in the usual position.

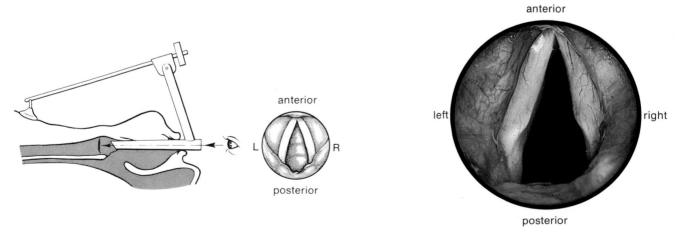

Example VI: Direct laryngoscopy: The glottis during inspiration.

Diseases of the Ear

Diseases of the Auricle

Congenital Defects

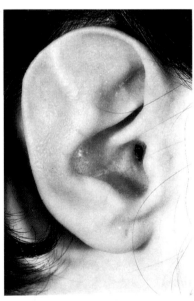

1

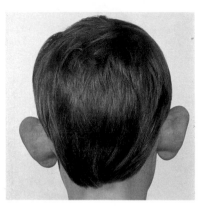

2

1–2 Outstanding ears

A cosmetically pleasing auricle is present when the concha is positioned at about 90° to the lateral surface of the head, the helix and anthelix are well formed, and there is a scapha-concha angle of 90°. The most common cause of protruding auricles as in this patient is lack of proper angulation between the scapha and the concha due to maldevelopment of the anthelix or excessive concavity of the concha. Protruding ears can cause severe psychologic problems for the patient and should be corrected surgically.

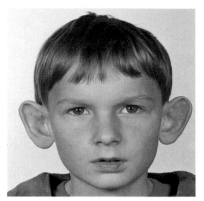

3

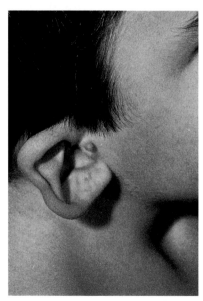

4

3 Auricular deformity

There is an abnormal fold between the helix and anthelix.

4 "Lop" ear

There is an additional auricular appendage on the tragus. The child has the Klippel-Feil syndrome.

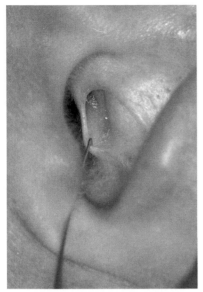

5 Congenital deformity of external canal, left
There is an incomplete septum in the external auditory canal. The posterior aperture ends in a blind pocket. The anterior meatus leads to a normal tympanic membrane through a narrow external auditory canal. – At times, a complete septum extends to the level of the tympanic membrane and forms a double external canal. In congenital deformities similar to this there are often other associated defects of the middle ear. Tomography is indicated to evaluate middle ear and ossicular abnormalities.

5

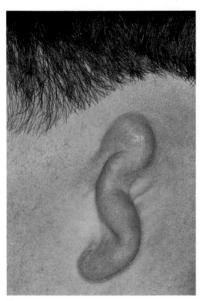

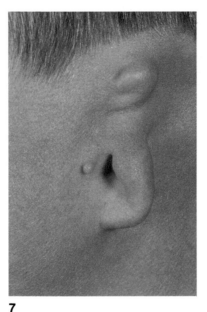

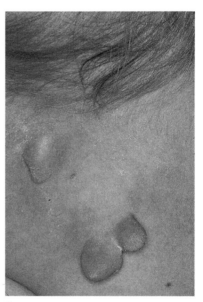

6   **7**   **8**

6–8 Congenital microtia and anotia
Congenital microtia and anotia are frequently associated with anomalies of the middle and inner ear and with facial anomalies such as mandibular facial dysostosis. – In microtia of the first degree the anatomical parts of the auricle are recognizable. With second degree microtia, Figs **6, 7,** the auricle is a rudimentary, vertical, slightly curved ridge. In these patients there was as-sociated atresia of the external canal and middle ear with severe deafness. – Third-degree microtia, Fig. **8,** is characterized by complete anotia or, as in this patient, by one or more small cutaneous or chondrocutaneous nodules. There is atresia of the external canal, and the only trace of the external canal is a small pit between the two nodules.

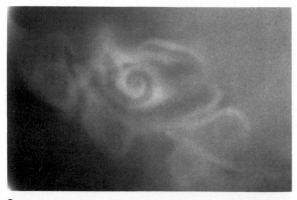

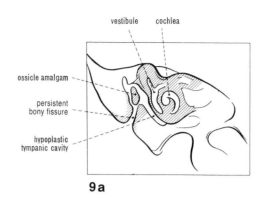

9a

9

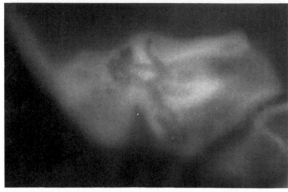

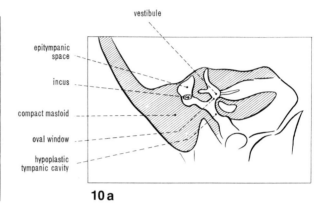

10a

10

9 Atresia of the right external auditory canal
In congenital atresias of the auricles tomography provides information about the development of the external auditory canal, the middle ear, the ossicles and the inner ear. – Frontal tomogram showing a persistent small fissure between the dysplastic tympanic bone and the mastoid, hypoplasia of the tympanic cavity, and a single amalgam of the ossicles. Normal inner ear structures.

10 Atresia of the right external auditory canal
Frontal tomogram showing complete agenesis of the external auditory canal and hypoplasia of the tympanic cavity. Normal inner ear structures.

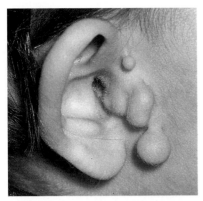

11

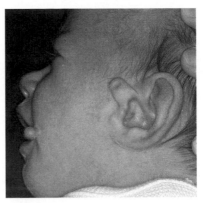

12

11–12 Auricular appendages, polyotia
Auricular appendages are ectodermal chondrocutaneous hyperplasias which, in many cases, are due to autosomal dominance with variable penetration. Most appendages occur in the preauricular area, Fig. **11**. – With disturbances in the fusion between the maxillary and mandibular processes of the first branchial arch, appendages can occur anywhere between the preauricular area and the corner of the mouth as in Fig. **12**.

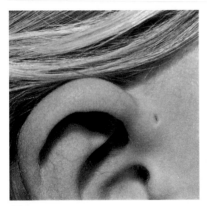

13

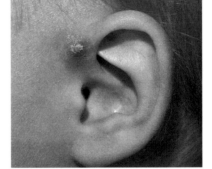

14

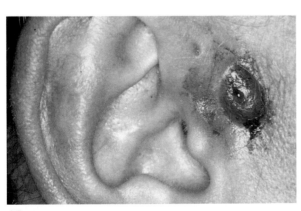

15

13–15 Congenital fistulae occur just anterior to the helix and arise from defects in fusion of the auricular hillocks of the first branchial groove. They are frequently bilateral. When not infected, a preauricular fistula appears as a small discrete pit at the anterior margin of the helix, Fig. **13**. – **Preauricular fistulae** are lined with stratified squamous epithelium, contain skin appendages, and may be short and end blindly or be several centimeters long and extensively branched. – When infected, preauricular cysts become reddened and swollen and suppurate, Figs **14** and **15**. Fistulae which become infected repeatedly should be removed surgically; it is important to excise all of the extensions of the lesion.

Trauma

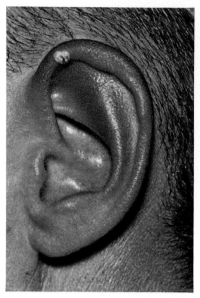

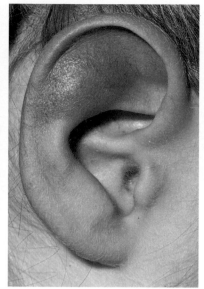

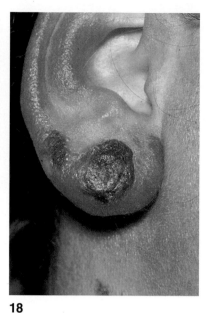

16   **17**   **18**

16 Painful nodule of the ear (nodulus helici chronica)
This condition is characterized by a tender ear nodule, histological examination of which reveals hyperkeratosis superimposed upon an often barely noticeable necrosis of the underlying cartilage.

17 Lymphadenosis benigna cutis
Following an insect bite there is a reactive proliferation of the lymphoreticular tissue of the derma in the upper portion of the auricle.

18 Lupoid granuloma of the lobule
This lesion occurred following piercing of the lobule for earrings.

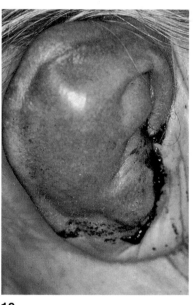

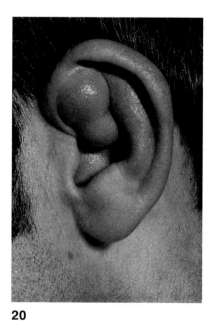

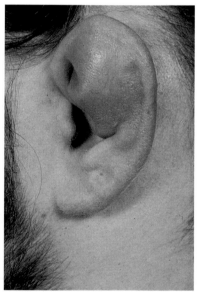

19   **20**   **21**

19 Othematoma
There is a fresh othematoma of the entire auricle following recent severe trauma.

20 Othematoma
This hematoma following tangential trauma, which occurred thirteen days before, is swollen and tense.

21 Organized othematoma
This patient is a stevedore who injured his ear many months earlier. An othematoma developed but was not treated. The hematoma has organized and caused this chronic deformity.

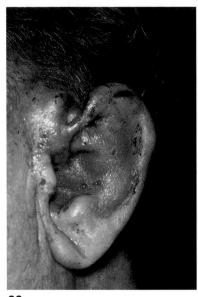

22

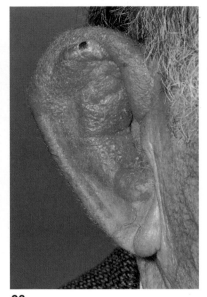

23

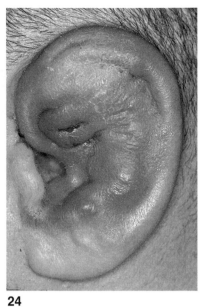

24

22 Post-traumatic cellulitis and perichondritis
Injury was sustained several days earlier in the course of a drunken brawl. The auricle was torn from its upper attachment and secondary infection ensued.

23 Perichondritis of the auricle
Chronic perichondritis of the auricle was caused by an erosion of the skin of the upper margin of the helix.

24 Perichondritis of the auricle
This perichondritis followed an endaural incision and tympanoplasty. Antibiotic therapy and incision were unsuccessful in relieving the perichondritis.

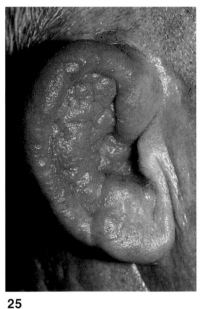

25

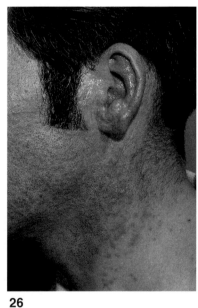

26

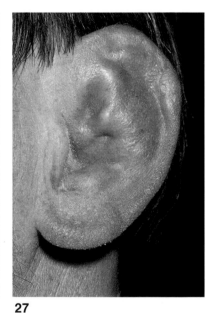

27

25 Chronic relapsing polychondritis
Chronic relapsing polychondritis of the auricle is associated with episodes of elevated temperature and inflammation of the nasal and tracheal cartilages as well as of the joints of the extremities.

26 Perichondritis, allergic
This allergic perichondritis followed use of chloramphenicol ear drops. The adjacent preauricular and neck skin are involved.

27 Cauliflower ear
This auricular deformity is the end stage of a chronic perichondritis.

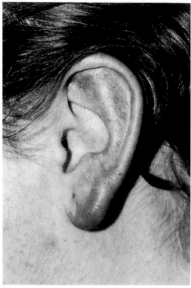

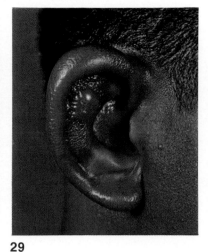

29

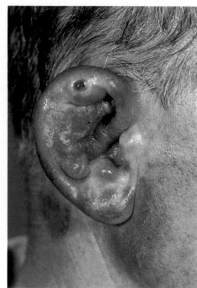

28

30

28 Frostbite of the auricle
Frostbite follows exposure to extreme cold. There is reddish blue discoloration and swelling of the affected skin.

29 Frostbite of the auricle
Two hours following exposure to extreme cold, the auricle became swollen and vesicles appeared. Immediately

after exposure the patient noted numbness of the ears, but pain and tenderness soon followed. Conservative treatment resulted in complete resolution.

30 Perichondritis following frostbite
This lesion, too, followed exposure of the uncovered auricles to extreme cold. There is a severe, infected perichondritis with ulceration on the helix margin.

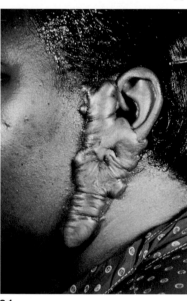

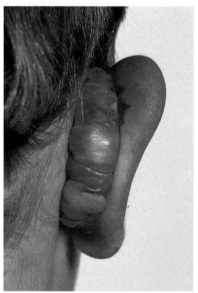

31

32

31 Keloid formation
These keloids originated as a result of piercing the lobule for earrings. Several operations were attempted to remove the original keloid, but each successive procedure produced more keloid and resulted in this extensive lesion. – While there is a strong tendency to keloid formation in those races with pigmented skin, keloid also occurs among whites.

32 Keloid
This keloid occurred in the postauricular scar of an otoplasty. The left ear was similarly affected.

Inflammatory and Metabolic Reactions of the Auricle

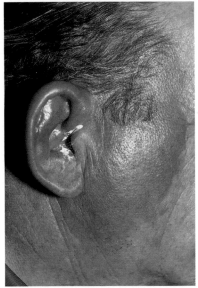

33

33 Bullous erysipelas of the auricle
There is a vesicular eruption of the auricle associated with an erythematous inflammation of the skin of the face. The onset occurred with a severe systemic reaction of chills, fever, malaise, involvement of the regional lymph nodes, and severe headache. The streptococcal infection was the result of a superficial abrasion of the skin of the auricle.

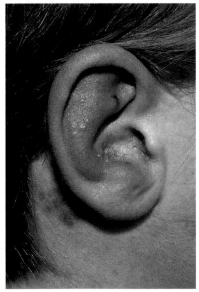

34

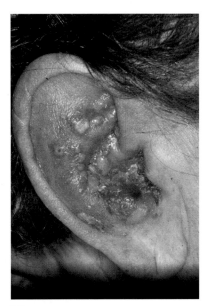

35

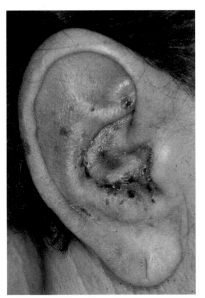

36

34 Herpes zoster oticus with Ramsey-Hunt syndrome
Five days previously there was a sudden onset of severe earache, a vesicular eruption on the auricle, and an ipsilateral peripheral facial nerve paralysis. There was an accompanying viral meningoencephalitis, vertigo, and sensorineural deafness.

35 Herpes zoster oticus
The patient had complained of a severe earache on the right side of three days' duration. There was a vesicular

eruption on the external ear and peripheral facial paresis; meningoencephalitis ensued. The vestibular reaction was decreased, and there was sensorineural deafness on the involved side (see Fig. **36**).

36 Herpes zoster oticus
Same ear shown in Fig. **35**. In this view, taken ten days later, multiple brownish yellow and black crusts have formed as the herpetic lesions have undergone resolution.

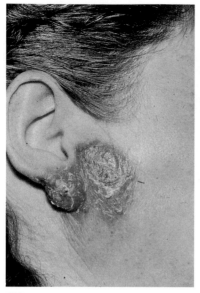

37

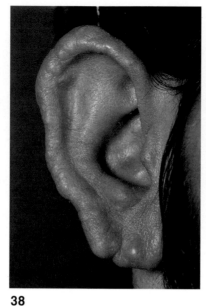

38

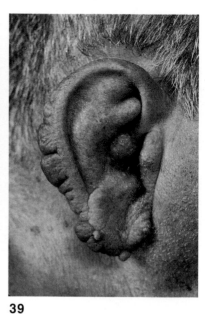

39

37 Lupus vulgaris of the ear lobe
The preauricular skin is affected along with that of the lobe. Differentiation from Boeck's sarcoid is based on the bluish red color of sarcoid and the brownish red color of lupus. By pressing a glass slide firmly on the lesion, one can observe the typical lupus spots with their apple jelly color. Biopsy is frequently necessary to establish a diagnosis.

38 Leprosy of the auricle
This is the appearance of lepromatous leprosy involving the auricle. Mycobacterium leprae can be demonstrated in the lesions, see Figs **373, 444** and **846**.

39 Fissured enlargement of the external ear
An aural as well as postauricular discharge in association with chronic suppurative otitis media resulted in perichondritis with fissuring and a papillary-like excrescence of the auricle.

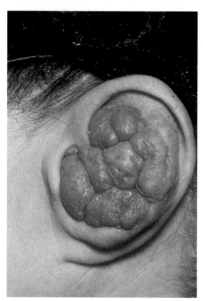

40

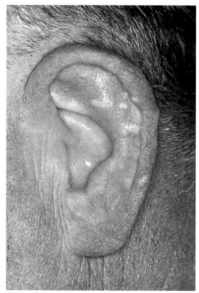

41

40 Elephantiasis
This soft compressible mass had been developing in this 58-year-old female patient for 30 years. It was characterized by hyperplastic changes in the skin and subcutaneous tissues as the result of recurrent cellulitis, which produced a blockage of lymphatic and venous channels.

41 Gouty tophi of the auricle
Several white-yellow nodules are present on the margin of the helix and anthelix. They are slightly protuberant and contain a greasy, chalky substance made up of urate or sodium biurate crystals.

Tumors

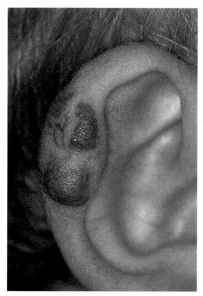

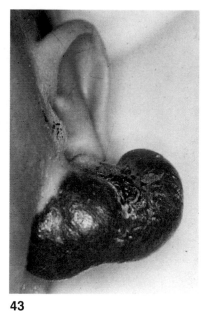

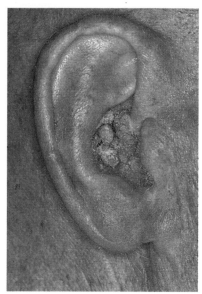

42

43

44

42 Congenital hemangioma of auricle
The lesion lies on the helix.

43 Cavernous hemangioma
The lesion involves the ear lobule, and there is an ulceration in the center of the lesion. This child had multiple small hemangiomas of the hands and arms.

44 Senile keratois of the auricle
Senile keratotic lesions should be removed surgically, since a transition to basal cell or squamous cell carcinoma is not infrequent; a histological section should be available for study.

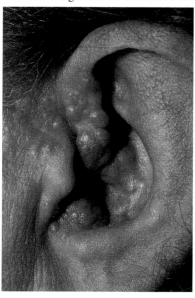

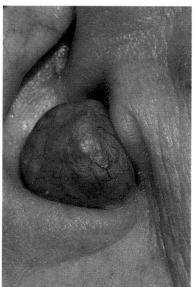

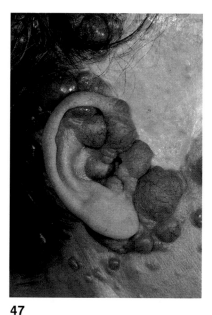

45

46

47

45 Adenoid basal cell epithelioma
There is an extensive adenoid cystic basal cell epithelioma of the cavum concha and intertragal notch.

46 Apocrine adenoma of the cylindromatous type
The singular lesion arises in the cavum concha. This lesion histologically is not identical with adenoid cystic carcinomas also known as cylindromas which involve the salivary glands.

47 Multiple apocrine adenomas of the cylindromatous type
These lesions also known as turban tumors are of the multiple and familiar type. These lesions rarely ulcerate or become malignant.

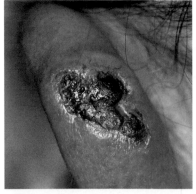

48

48 Ulcerated basal cell carcinoma
There is a basal cell carcinoma on the posterior aspect of the helix. The margin of the ulcerated lesion is raised and reddened.

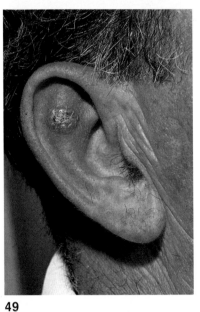

49

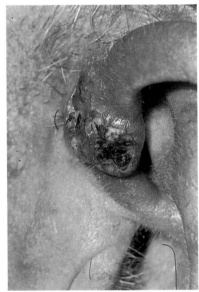

50

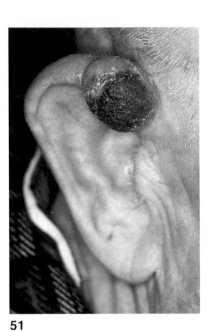

51

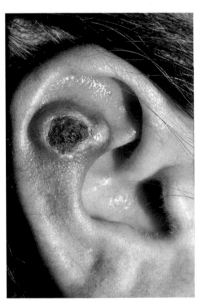

52

49–52 Squamous cell carcinomas resembling keratoacanthoma
Each of the lesions in Figs **49–52** clinically resemble keratoacanthoma but, in each case, biopsy showed squamous cell carcinoma. Keratoacanthoma is a rare lesion, difficult to diagnose, and biopsy and careful observation are necessary for any case in which this diagnosis is made.

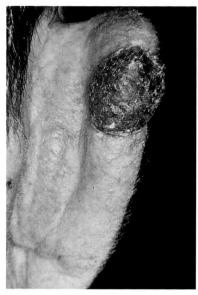

53

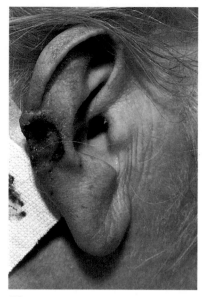

54

53 Squamous cell carcinoma of helix
There is an early squamous cell carcinoma occurring in an area of senile atrophy of the skin of the helix.

54 Squamous cell carcinoma
There is a crusted, ulcerated carcinoma on the helix extending to the anthelix

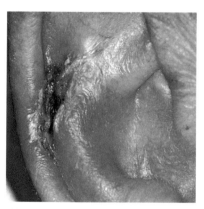

55

55 Squamous cell carcinoma
An ulcerated carcinoma lies between the helix and anthelix.

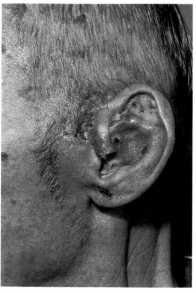

56

56 Squamous cell carcinoma
This lesion of the auricle and preauricular area was misdiagnosed and treated for several months with topical ointment.

The Diagnosis and Differential Diagnosis of Malignant Melanomas

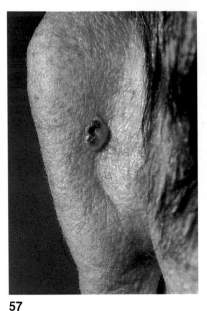

57

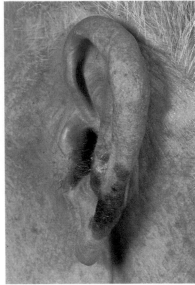

58

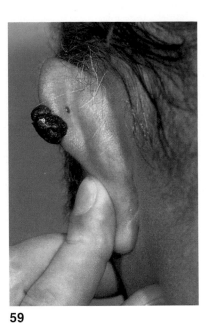

59

57 Pigmented basal cell carcinoma
There is a small, nodular pigmented lesion on the posterior surface of the auricle. The blue-black pigment suggests melanoma, but excisional biopsy proved the lesion to be a pigmented basal cell carcinoma.

58 Lentigo maligna
This disorder is also known as melanosis circumscripta preblastomatosa. Lentigo maligna is considered to be a malignant melanoma in situ. This small brown lesion on

the helix enlarged slowly and was treated by partial auriculectomy. Untreated lentigo maligna will undergo degeneration into a malignant melanoma.

59 Malignant melanoma
There is a typical, nodular, deeply pigmented malignant melanoma on the helix margin. There is a small cutaneous metastasis on the postauricular surface. Diagnosis proven by biopsy.

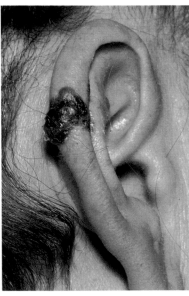

60

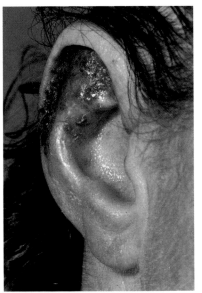

61

60 Malignant melanoma
There is a partially pigmented, ulcerated lesion on the helix margin. The lesion was pruritic and bled easily when scratched. Diagnosis proven by biopsy.

61 Malignant melanoma
In this case there was a sudden increase in growth during the year of a small, pinhead-sized pigmented mole of the auricle. The lesion became a large, partially pigmented, ulcerated and crusted malignant melanoma.

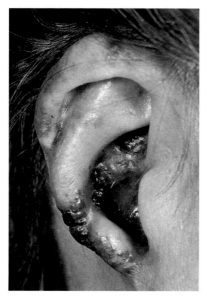

62

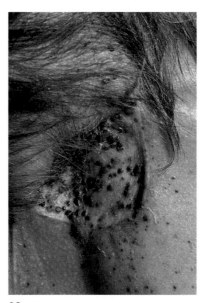

63

62 Malignant melanoma, diffuse
The malignant melanoma has infiltrated extensively and caused severe deformity and pigmentation of the auricle.

63 Malignant melanoma, diffuse, same patient as Fig. 62
The auricle in Fig. **62** was widely excised and the surgical defect covered with a split skin graft. Three weeks postoperatively, extensive local and metastatic dissemination occurred.

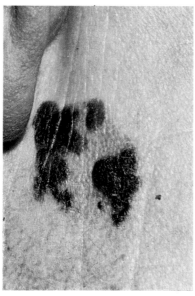

64

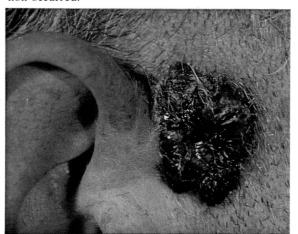

65

64 Malignant melanoma
This irregular, nodular melanoma lies in a lentigo maligna lesion, which in turn arose from a pigmented mole present since birth. The auricle is at the left.

65 Malignant melanoma
There is an extensive blue-black malignant melanoma extending from the helix crus to the preauricular skin. Sometimes malignant melanomas may be nonpigmented. They metastasize widely and early. Signs of malignant change from a benign skin lesion to a malignant melanoma include sudden increase in size, deepening pigmentation, oozing, itching, bleeding, or crusting of a previously harmless-appearing mole.

Diseases of the External Auditory Canal; Foreign Bodies

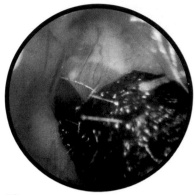

66

66 Cerumen
There is a round mass of cerumen in the external canal. The cerumen does not occlude the canal and the tympanic membrane is visible superiorly. Since the canal was not completely occluded the patient noted no symptoms.

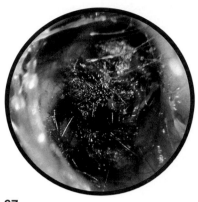

67

67 Cerumen
Cerumen occludes the external canal completely, causing hearing loss and a sense of fullness in the affected ear.

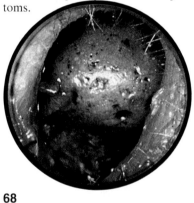

68   **69**

68 Foreign body, external canal, left
There is a stone wedged tightly in the external canal of this child. The canal lumen is completely occluded.

69 Foreign body, external canal, left
A pearl bead lies in this child's canal.

70

70 Foreign body, matchstick, left
This patient tried to scratch his ear with a matchstick and broke off a piece of the match which lodged in the canal. He has abraded the canal where there is a bit of blood. There is a bit of cerumen superiorly.

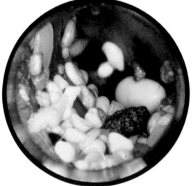

71

71 Foreign bodies, coral sand, left
This patient noted fullness in his ears following body surfing at a beach in Hawaii.

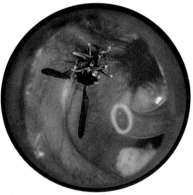

72

72 Foreign body, insect, right
A polyethylene tube is present from previous treatment of serous otitis media.

Infections

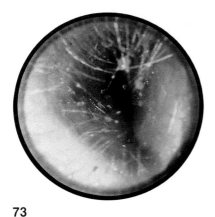

73

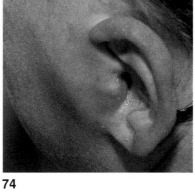

74

73 Acute external otitis, right
There is acute cellulitis of the external auditory canal with inflammation, edema, and severe tenderness of the canal. The concentric swelling of the skin of the canal narrows the lumen of the canal to one-fourth its normal size.

74 Furunculosis external canal, left
There is a swollen, reddened, painful furuncle involving the tragus and the anterior wall of the external meatus. There is a regional lymphadenitis in the parotid area.

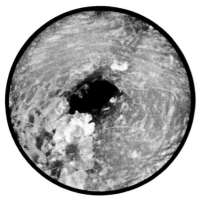

75 Chronic external otitis, left
For many years this patient had chronic recurrent external otitis. The skin of the external auditory canal is thickened and fibrosed, decreasing the lumen of the canal to 5 to 10 percent of its normal size.

75

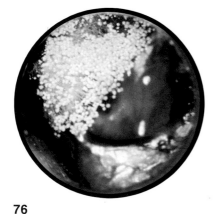

76

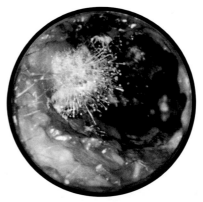

77

76 Otomycosis, external auditory canal, right
The posterior half of the external auditory canal is filled with a greenish-yellow fungus. The round sporangia are clearly evident growing at the ends of the white mycelia. Note the purulent discharge in the inferior portion of the canal.

77 Otomycosis in a radical mastoidectomy cavity, right
Growing in the lumen of the mastoidectomy cavity is this mass of fungus. The fungi are clearly visible against the dark and light purple background of the gentian violet applied earlier to the mastoid cavity.

Exostoses

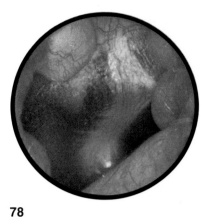

78

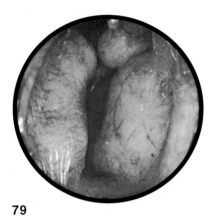

79

78 Multiple exostoses, external auditory canal, right
Four small, smooth, rounded protuberances lie lateral to the drum. These exostoses arise from the tympanic annulus. The bony external canal lies to the right inferiorly; the pars tensa is normal.

79 Severe exostoses, external auditory canal, left
This patient had a history of having done a good deal of swimming in the past. Approximately 85 percent of the lumen of the external auditory canal is occluded by large, broad-based exostoses. The small lumen can easily become occluded with cerumen and epithelial debris.

Malignant Tumors

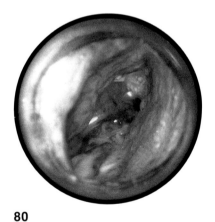

80

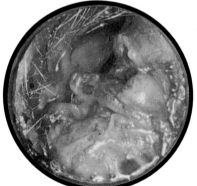

81

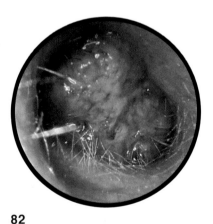

82

80 Squamous cell carcinoma, external auditory canal, right
This patient had a chronic, weeping external otitis of many years' duration. A polyp had developed three years previously, but biopsy was negative. The patient was not seen until he returned with the external auditory canal filled with the granular lesions which occupy the circumference of the cartilaginous and bony canal and extend to the tympanic membrane. Biopsy showed squamous cell carcinoma. Tomography showed erosion of bone adjacent to the descending facial nerve.

81 Squamous cell carcinoma, external auditory canal, right
A granulomatous mass fills the lumen of the external canal. Biopsy showed malignancy and a wide excision was performed. This lesion bled easily on contact.

82 Squamous cell carcinoma, external auditory canal, left
The patient complained for two months of a bloody discharge and pain, especially when chewing. The granular, red mass fills the external canal almost completely.

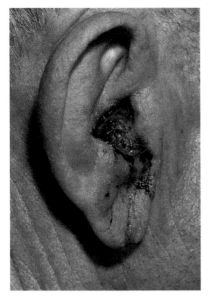

83

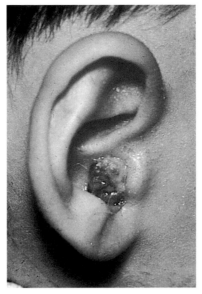

84

83 Squamous cell carcinoma, external canal, right
For many years this 78-year-old patient noted suppurative discharge and deafness in his right ear. Over a period of a few weeks this polyp appeared in the meatus. The polyp bled easily on contact and biopsy showed squamous cell carcinoma.

84 Fibromyxosarcoma
This 2-year-old male presented with right facial paralysis of three weeks' duration. In addition there was a slight, diffuse, nontender swelling anterior and superior to the right auricle extending to the external canal. The meatus was filled with a friable granular mass identified as a fibromyxosarcoma. The tumor grew rapidly and the child succumbed when intracranial extension occurred. In young children such granular or polypoid tissue is frequently associated with Hand-Schüller-Christian disease or is sarcomatous in character, possibly of middle ear origin.

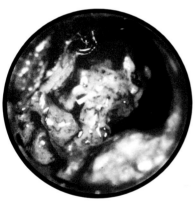

85

85 Carcinoma middle ear and mastoid, post-radical mastoidectomy, right
A granulomatous carcinoma protrudes from an old radical mastoidectomy cavity into the external auditory canal. – Carcinomatous degeneration of chronic suppurating ears is very rare, but the otologist must always be alert and must biopsy suspicious polypoid ear lesions.

Diseases of the Middle Ear and Mastoid

Anatomy of the Middle Ear and Mastoid

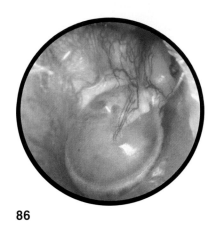

86

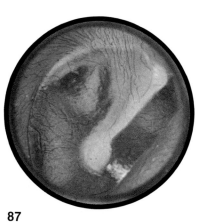

87

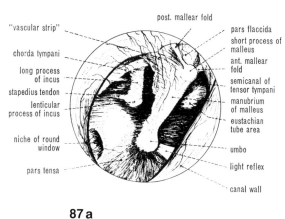

87a

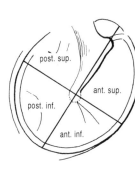

87b

86 Tympanic membrane, right
This is the view of a tympanic membrane seen with the ear endoscope. There is a slight reactive hyperemia of the blood vessels running along the manubrium of the malleus, and a slight retraction of the posterosuperior quadrant of the membrane. The telescope offers a wide field view of the entire tympanic membrane, the annulus, and a portion of the external auditory canal.

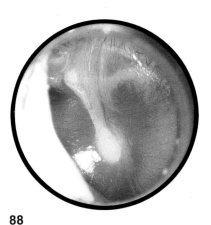

88

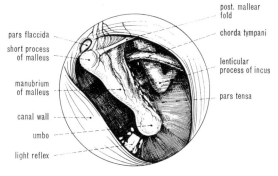

88a

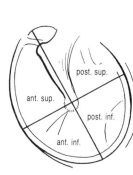

88b

87 Normal tympanic membrane, right
The tympanic membrane is almost transparent. – Structures visible through the membrane in the posterior portion of the middle ear are: the chorda tympani, the long process of the incus, the oval window niche, the promontory, and the round window niche. Anterosuperiorly, the canal for the tensor tympani and the opening of the eustachian tube are apparent through the membrane.

88 Normal tympanic membrane, left
The small pars flaccida lies above the short process of the malleus. The chorda tympani arches across the upper part of the posterosuperior quadrant. The faint whitish area posterosuperiorly is the lenticular process of the incus. – The gray-white color of this tympanic membrane is more normal than the darker color of the almost transparent tympanic membrane in Fig **87. Quadrants of the tympanic membrane** (Figs. **87b, 88b**).

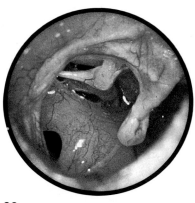

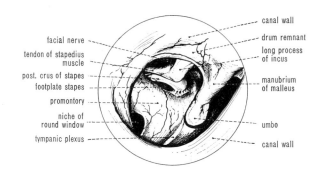

canal wall
facial nerve
drum remnant
tendon of stapedius muscle
long process of incus
post. crus of stapes
footplate stapes
manubrium of malleus
promontory
niche of round window
umbo
tympanic plexus
canal wall

89

89 a

89 Middle ear structures exposed by large central perforation, right
A small portion of the posterosuperior pars tensa re-

mains exposing the: tympanic plexus, promontory, oval and round window niches, incus long process, stapedius tendon, stapes crura, and the facial nerve.

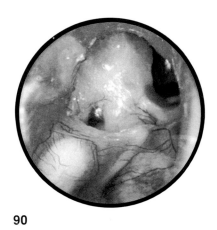

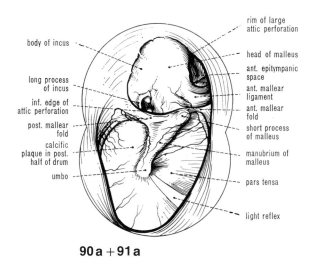

rim of large attic perforation
body of incus
head of malleus
ant. epitympanic space
long process of incus
ant. mallear ligament
inf. edge of attic perforation
ant. mallear fold
post. mallear fold
short process of malleus
calcific plaque in post. half of drum
manubrium of malleus
umbo
pars tensa
light reflex

90

90a + 91a

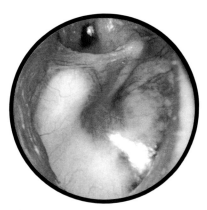

91

90 Large epitympanic slough, right
An epitympanic cholesteatoma has sloughed the notch of Rivinus and lateral epitympanic wall to expose the head of the malleus and the anterior portion of the body of the incus. The long process of the incus extends into the mesotympanum. The medial wall of the cholesteatoma sac stretches between the anterior surface of the malleus head and the anterior wall of the epitympanum.

91 Same ear as Fig. 90
When the otoscope is directed inferiorly, tympanosclerotic deposits within the posterior half of the pars tensa are apparent. The inferior margin of the epitympanic perforation is the elongated posterior tympanomallear fold. The neck of the malleus and long process of the incus appear above the posterior tympanomallear fold. – The diagram was made by superimposing the photographs.

Anatomy of the Eustachian Tube

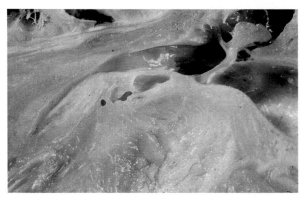

92

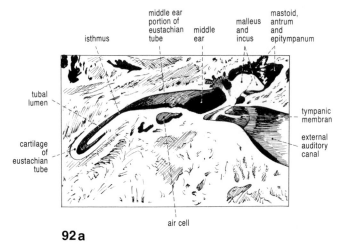

92a

92 Cross section of temporal bone, Stenvers plane, normal, left

This section shows the bony eustachian tube from the beginning of the cartilaginous portion to the middle ear. The lower half of the tympanic membrane lies below sections of the malleus and incus. The external auditory canal and mastoid antrum extend laterally.

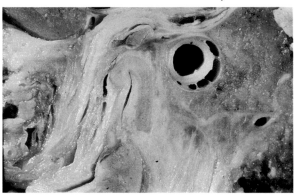

93

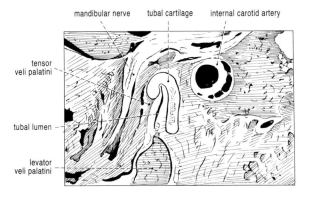

93a

93 Axial cross section of temporal bone through the cartilaginous portion of eustachian tube, right

The inverted J-shaped cartilage of the eustachian tube lies between the internal carotid artery and the mandibular branch of the fifth cranial nerve. The tensor veli palatini muscle attaches to the hook of the cartilage. The levator veli palatini muscle lies below the narrow, elongated lumen of the eustachian tube. The mandibular branch of the fifth cranial nerve descends lateral to the tube.

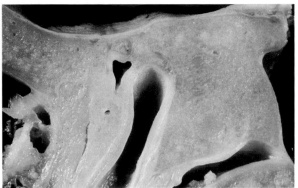

94

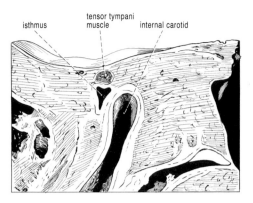

94a

94 Axial cross section of temporal bone at the level of the isthmus of the eustachian tube, right

The isthmus of the eustachian tube lies lateral to the internal carotid artery.

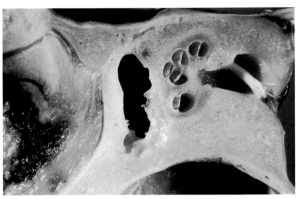

95

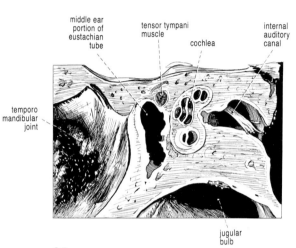

95a

95 Axial cross section of temporal bone through the middle ear portion of the eustachian tube, right

The widened middle ear portion of the eustachian tube is bounded medially by the cochlea and laterally by the tympanic bone and temporomandibular joint.

Radiography of the Ear

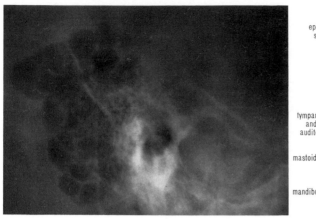

96

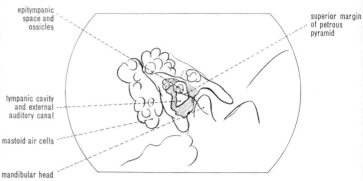

96 a

96 Normal mastoid, right
Schüller's projection of a normal mastoid obtained with a 30-degree cephalocaudal angulation of the x-ray beam. Note that the epitympanic space with the ossicles is visible.

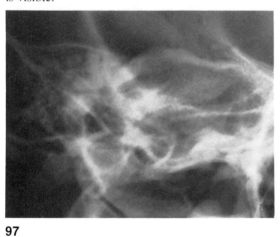

97

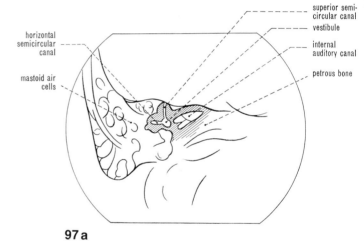

97 a

97 Normal mastoid and petrous pyramid, Stenvers projection

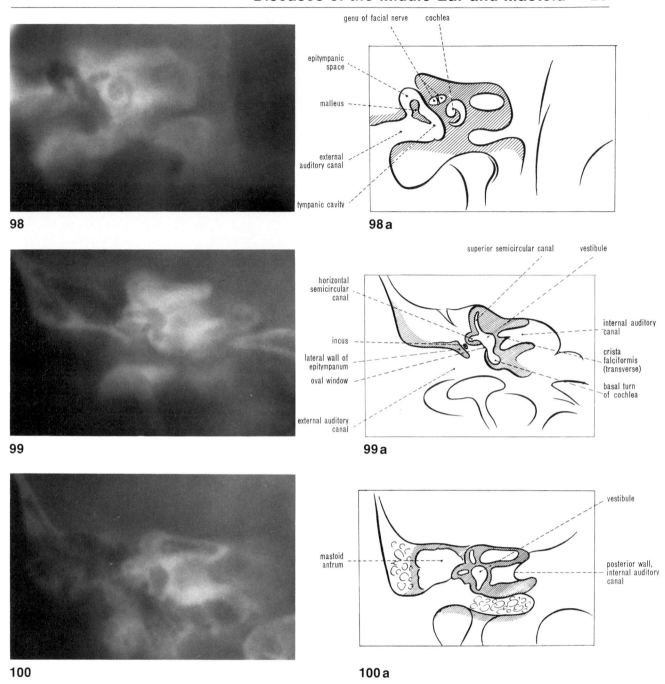

98   Frontal tomogram of a normal right ear

99   Frontal tomogram of a normal right ear obtained
     5 mm posterior to the view seen in Fig. 98

100 Frontal tomogram of a normal right ear obtained
     3 mm posterior to the view seen in Fig. 99

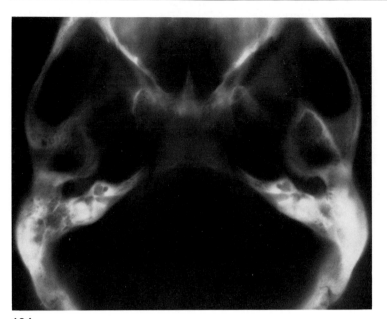

101

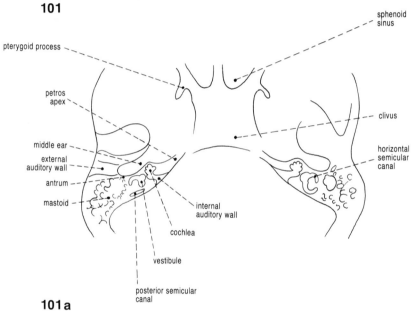

sphenoid
sinus

pterygoid process

petros
apex

clivus

middle ear

external
auditory wall

antrum

mastoid

horizontal
semicular
canal

internal
auditory wall

cochlea

vestibule

posterior semicular
canal

101a

**101 Horizontal tomogram of the base of a normal skull
at the level of the middle and inner ears**

Traumatic Lesions of the Tympanic Membrane and Temporal Bone

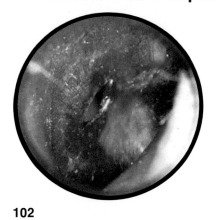

102

102 Traumatic rupture of tympanic membrane, right
There is a rupture of the posterosuperior quadrant of the hemorrhagic tympanic membrane. The red color of the extravasated blood in the tympanic membrane is evidence of the recent trauma, a slap to the ear. The lesion healed spontaneously.

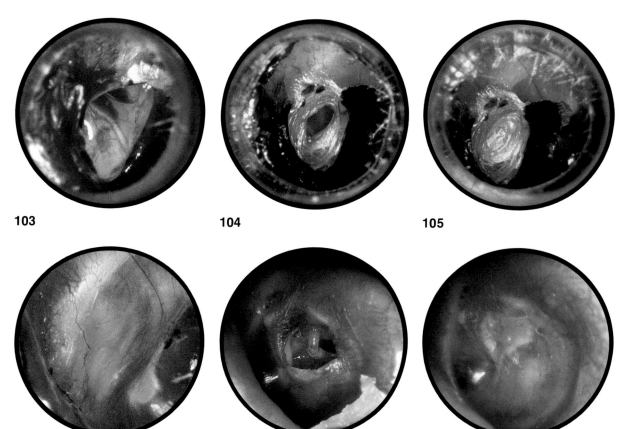

103   **104**   **105**

106   **107**   **108**

103 Traumatic perforation of tympanic membrane with spontaneous healing, right
The patient accidentally ruptured his tympanic membrane with a Q-tip a few hours previously. There is a large perforation of the posterior half of the tympanic membrane. The lenticular process is exposed superiorly.

104 Same ear as Figs 103, 105, and 106
One month after the accident the perforation has decreased in size. A circular crust lies on the margin of the perforation.

105 Same ear as Figs 103, 104, and 106
Two months later, the concentric rings in the crust indicate the method of healing.

106 Same ear as Figs 103, 104, and 105
The crust in Fig. **105** has been lifted out of the external canal to reveal the healed tympanic membrane.

107 Traumatic perforation, tympanic membrane, left
The perforation caused by a blow to the ear exposes the incudostapedial joint.

108 Same ear as Fig. 107
Following closure of the perforation five weeks earlier with a fibrous adhesive in current use in Europe, the perforation has healed.

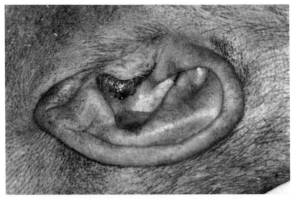

109

109 Cerebrospinal fluid otorrhea, left ear
This 69-year-old male fell while drunk and sustained radiographically proved transverse and longitudinal fractures of the left temporal bone. There was a contused laceration of the left forehead, spontaneous second-degree nystagmus to the right, and a severe left hearing loss. There was a hematotympanum. As seen here there were periauricular hematomas, and the cerebrospinal fluid otorrhea was evident as fluid pooled in the cavum conchae when the patient was supine.

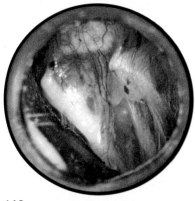

110

110 Basal skull fracture involving bony external auditory canal, left
There is a notch in the posterosuperior bony sulcus tympanicus caused by a basal fracture which displaced the fragments. The skull fracture occurred several months earlier. The scarred tympanic membrane is a residue of the rupture of the tympanic membrane which occurred at the time of injury. Bleeding from the ear which often occurs with basal skull fractures is caused by rupture of the skin of the external auditory canal and of the tympanic membrane. When the fracture involves the tegmen of the mastoid and adjacent dura, there is cerebrospinal otorrhea.

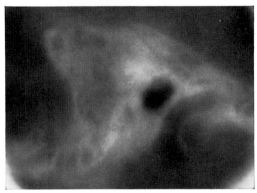

111

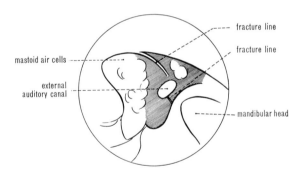

111a

111 Longitudinal basal skull fracture, lateral tomogram, right
The tomogram shows the fracture line extending from the mastoid tegmen to the posterosuperior margin of the external auditory canal. The fracture line extends across to the anteroinferior margin of the external canal. – Fig. 110 shows the otoscopic appearance of such a fracture several months after injury.

Secretory Otitis Media

Other terms: Serous otitis media, Otitis media with effusion, Middle ear effusion, Mucoid otitis media, Chronic otitis media with effusion, Catarrhal otitis media, Glue ear.

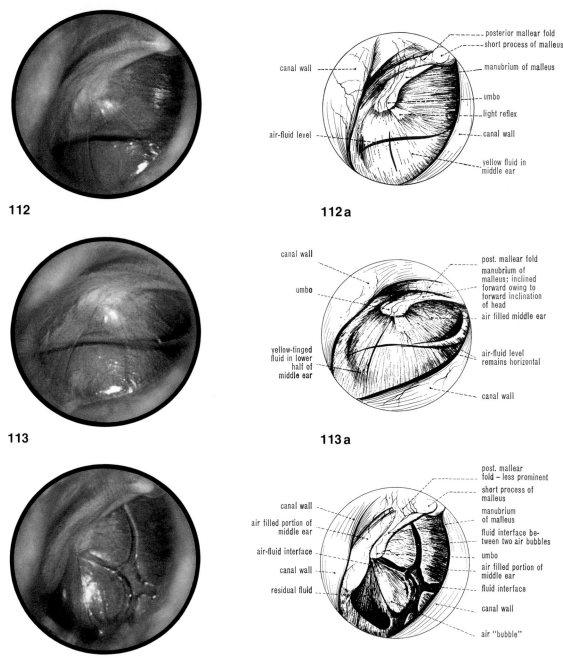

112

112a
- posterior mallear fold
- short process of malleus
- manubrium of malleus
- canal wall
- umbo
- light reflex
- air-fluid level
- canal wall
- yellow fluid in middle ear

113

113a
- canal wall
- umbo
- post. mallear fold
- manubrium of malleus; inclined forward owing to forward inclination of head
- air filled middle ear
- air-fluid level remains horizontal
- yellow-tinged fluid in lower half of middle ear
- canal wall

114

114a
- canal wall
- air filled portion of middle ear
- air-fluid interface
- canal wall
- residual fluid
- post. mallear fold – less prominent
- short process of malleus
- manubrium of malleus
- fluid interface between two air bubbles
- umbo
- air filled portion of middle ear
- fluid interface
- canal wall
- air "bubble"

112 Secretory otitis media, horizontal fluid level, right
A small amount of yellow serous fluid lies in the hypotympanum below the umbo. The horizontal, black, refractile line is the air-fluid interface. The malleus short process and the posterior malleus fold are prominent because of slight inward retraction of the tympanic membrane.

113 Same ear as Figs 112 and 114
To demonstrate the fluid nature of the middle ear secretion, the patient's head is rotated forward approximately 40°, but the air fluid interface remains horizontal.

114 Same ear as Figs 112 and 113, following politzerization
Insufflation of air by politzerization disperses the fluid into a series of large air bubbles within the middle ear.

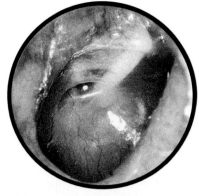

115

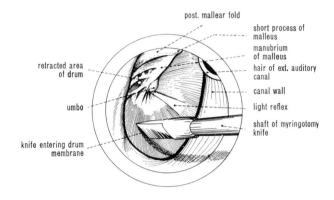

canal wall

folds of drum due to localized retraction

entire middle ear filled with fluid

post. mallear fold

short process of malleus

manubrium of malleus

umbo

canal wall

light reflex

115a

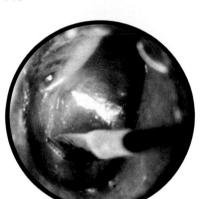

116

retracted area of drum

umbo

knife entering drum membrane

post. mallear fold

short process of malleus

manubrium of malleus

hair of ext. auditory canal

canal wall

light reflex

shaft of myringotomy knife

116a

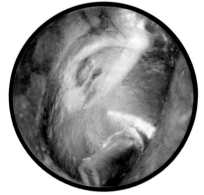

117

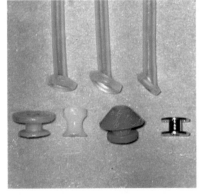

118

115 Secretory otitis media, myringotomy and polyethylene tube insertion, right

The entire middle ear is filled with a deep amber-colored serous fluid. The short process and the posterior mallear fold are prominent because of the medial retraction of the tympanic membrane. There are two or three folds in the posterosuperior quadrant due to relatively more retraction of less-resistant areas of the membrane. The malleus handle appears chalky in relation to the color of the serous fluid.

116 Myringotomy, same ear as Figs 115 and 117

A myringotomy knife is piercing the tympanic membrane.

117 Status post myringotomy and intubation, same ear as Figs 115 and 116

Six weeks after myringotomy and insertion of a middle ear air vent, the middle ear has a normal, air-filled appearance. The posterior mallear fold is less prominent, and the retraction folds of the posterosuperior quadrant have disappeared. The polyethylene tube lies inferiorly.

118 Commonly used types of middle ear ventilation tubes

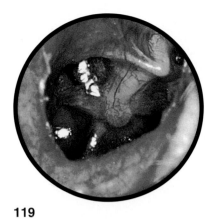

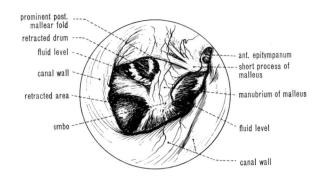

prominent post. mallear fold
retracted drum
fluid level
canal wall
retracted area
umbo

ant. epitympanum
short process of malleus
manubrium of malleus
fluid level
canal wall

119 **119a**

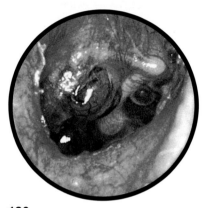

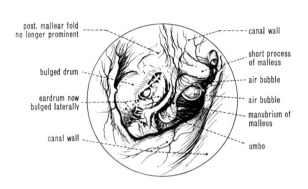

post. mallear fold no longer prominent
bulged drum
eardrum now bulged laterally
canal wall

canal wall
short process of malleus
air bubble
air bubble
manubrium of malleus
umbo

120 **120a**

119 Secretory otitis media, with moderate atelectasis, right

Except for the anterosuperior quadrant, the middle ear is filled with yellow-colored serous fluid. The horizontal air fluid interface stretching anteriorly from the umbo demonstrates the air-filled anterosuperior quadrant. – The posterior half of the middle ear is atelectatic and retracted medially. A thin strip of the pars tensa with a

middle fibrous layer stretches posteriorly from the umbo and resists retraction.

120 Secretory otitis media, same ear as Fig. 119

Insufflation of air into the middle ear by politzerization herniates the atrophic atelectatic areas of the posterior middle ear. The superior herniated area appears as an air-filled bleb.

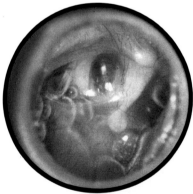

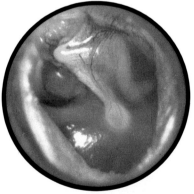

121 **122**

121 Secretory otitis media, right

The middle ear is partially filled with serous fluid and air. The menisci between the air bubbles and the fluid appear as curvilinear lines throughout all the quadrants of the tympanic membrane. Posterosuperiorly the tympanic membrane is retracted medially and lies in contact with the long process of the incus.

122 Secretory otitis media, left

Almost the entire middle ear is filled with a yellow-green serous fluid. There is an air bubble anterosuperiorly. The short process of the malleus and the posterior mallear fold are prominent. The long process of the incus and the head of the stapes and stapedius tendon are clearly visible in the posterior superior quadrant. As seen in this ear, visualization of the long process of the incus does not rule out serous otitis media.

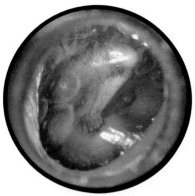

123

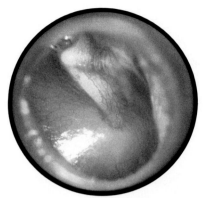

124

123 Secretory otitis media, right
The middle ear is partially filled with yellow serous fluid. Two air bubbles lie in the posterior portion of the middle ear. The menisci between the air-filled bubbles and the fluid-filled middle ear appear as curvilinear lines. There are three small air bubbles in the anterosuperior quadrant.

124 Secretory otitis media, left, same patient as Fig. 123
The entire middle ear of the opposite side of the patient in Fig. **123** is filled with a yellow-green fluid. The short process of the malleus is prominent. There are no air bubbles in this middle ear.

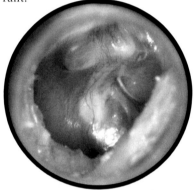

125

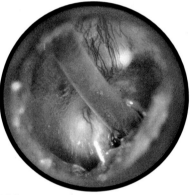

126

125 Secretory otitis media, right
The middle ear is partially filled with a yellow-bluish serous fluid. There are air bubbles in both superior quadrants.

126 Same ear as Fig. 125, following ventilation of the middle ear with an indwelling polyethylene tube
The middle ear is now air-filled and free of fluid. The tube is placed through the anterior quadrant and lies over the malleus handle.

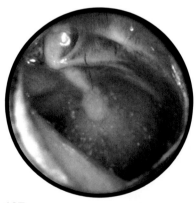

127

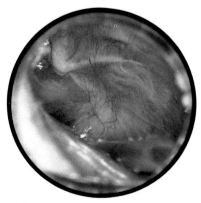

128

127 Secretory otitis media, left
The tympanic membrane has a yellow-blue cast due to serous fluid which fills the middle ear. The malleus handle is prominent. The posterior mallear fold stands out in strong relief and the pars flaccida is retracted.

128 Same ear as Fig. 127, following middle ear ventilation
Two months after treatment with a myringotomy and polyethylene tube, the middle ear is now air-filled and has a normal grayish appearance. The posterior mallear fold is much less prominent and the pars flaccida retraction is relieved. The polyethylene tube is seen inferiorly.

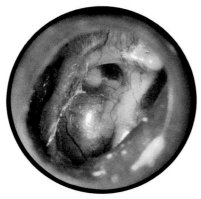

129

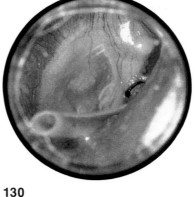

130

129 Secretory otitis media with atelectasis, right
The middle ear is filled with dark, yellow-green serous fluid. The atrophic posterior tympanic membrane is retracted medially and lies in contact with the head of the stapes and the long process of the incus.

130 Same ear as Fig. 129, following middle ear ventilation
Following treatment with an indwelling polyethylene middle ear ventilating tube, the ear shows relief of the retraction and expansion of the tympanic membrane to the normal position. The middle ear is now air-filled and has a normal gray appearance.

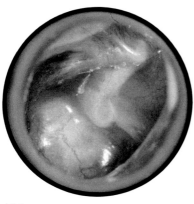

131

131 Secretory otitis media with atelectasis, right
The entire middle ear is filled with yellowish serous fluid. The posterior and part of the anteroinferior quadrants of the thin and atrophic membrane are retracted medially and lie in contact with the promontory. The posterior mallear fold is prominent.

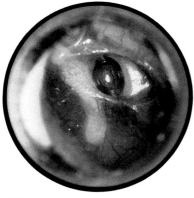

132

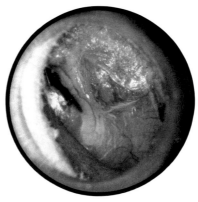

133

132 Secretory otitis media with atelectasis, six-year follow-up, left
The entire middle ear is filled with serous fluid, and there is atelectasis of the posterior superior quadrant of the middle ear. There is a deep retraction of an atrophic area of the tympanic membrane to the level of the long process of the incus. The posterior mallear fold is prominent. The patient was treated with indwelling polyethylene tube middle ear ventilation for about three

years, and the fluid and atelectasis disappeared. Following extrusion of the polyethylene tube, eustachian tube function and middle ear aeration were restored, and the tympanic membrane appearance returned to normal.

133 Same ear as Fig. 132, six years later
The ear shows the thin atrophic posterior superior quadrant of the tympanic membrane bulged slightly laterally in an air-filled middle ear.

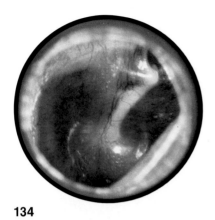

134

134 Secretory otitis media, hemotympanum, right
The entire middle ear is filled with a blue-colored serous fluid. The posterior mallear fold is prominent and the short process of the malleus is prominent. The malleus handle stands out in striking contrast to the bluish appearance of the middle ear. In all adults with secretory otitis or hemorrhagic secretory otitis, a careful nasopharyngeal examination is necessary to rule out tumors and malignancies as the cause of the eustachian malfunction. The fiberoptic telescope is useful in nasopharyngeal examination.

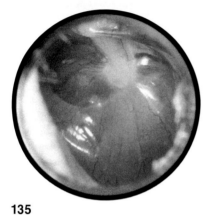

135

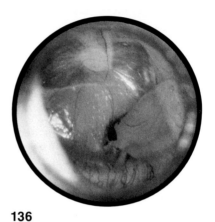

136

135 Serous otitis media, "glue type", left
The middle ear is partially filled with an opaque, pale yellow-colored fluid and the tympanic membrane is retracted. There is a curved interface anteriorly demarcating the gluey mucous inferiorly from air in the anterosuperior quadrant. The pale yellow, opaque color of the secretion within the middle ear strongly suggests gluey mucous.

136 Same ear as Fig. 135, post myringotomy
Immediately after the myringotomy, a portion of the gluey mucous has been aspirated from the middle ear. The thick strand of mucous lies inferiorly and stretches from the myringotomy into the external ear.

Acute Otitis Media and Mastoiditis

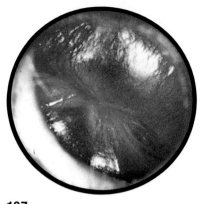 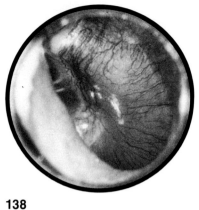 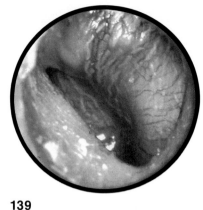

137 **138** **139**

137 Acute otitis media, left
This tympanic membrane is bulged laterally and is slightly hyperemic due to increased pressure and inflammatory exudate within the middle ear. The bulge of the membrane is most pronounced in the postero-superior quadrant. The blood vessels of the manubrium of the malleus and the pars flaccida are injected. This patient had earache, fever, and malaise caused by the infection.

138 Acute otitis media, left
This is an early stage of acute otitis media with moderate inflammation and lateral bulging of the tympanic membrane. The patient noted earache and fever.

139 Acute otitis media, left
The tympanic membrane is hyperemic and bulges laterally. There is injection of the vasculature along the malleus handle. The middle ear is filled with thick suppurative secretion and exudate which causes the whitish color of the tympanic membrane.

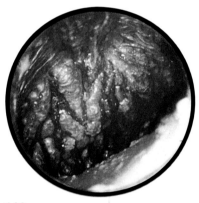 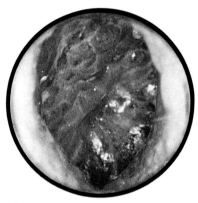

140 **141**

140 Acute otitis media, severe, right
The pars tensa is grossly inflamed, thickened, and bulged laterally. The superficial epithelium has begun to desquamate and has the appearance of alligator skin. The landmarks of the normal tympanic membrane, the malleus handle, umbo, and short process are obscured by the inflammation. There is seropurulent exudate within the middle ear under increased pressure.

141 Chronic myringitis, right
Chronic myringitis must be differentiated from acute otitis media, which it may resemble at times. In chronic myringitis there is a history of painless chronic discharge. The hearing is normal and the granular, nodular inflammation is confined to the tympanic membrane. There is no middle ear or systemic involvement, and the tympanic membrane is not perforated. – In this ear the umbo is the only visible landmark and a granular inflammation involves the posterior portion of the tympanic membrane.

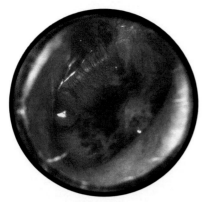

142

142 Acute otitis media, right
The entire pars tensa of the tympanic membrane is intensely injected and hemorrhagic. Exudate under increased pressure in the middle ear has produced a moderate lateral bulge of the membrane.

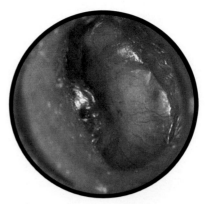

143

143 Acute otitis media, left
The tympanic membrane is hemorrhagic along the malleus handle and in the pars flaccida region. The membrane bulges laterally, due to secretion and exudate within the middle ear, which is under increased pressure. The patient had an elevated temperature and experienced severe earache.

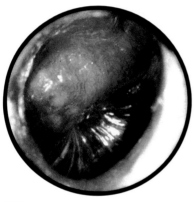

144

144 Acute otitis media with herniation of tympanic membrane, right
The posterior superior quadrant of the tympanic membrane is herniated laterally by exudate under increased pressure within the middle ear. The remaining portion of the tympanic membrane bulges laterally, but to a lesser degree. The malleus handle and a portion of the posterosuperior quadrant are injected. Herniation associated with inflammatory changes most probably accounts for dissolution of the middle fibrous layer of the posterosuperior quadrant of the tympanic membrane, as seen in Fig. **178**. Atrophic areas of the tympanic membrane make the ear susceptible to atelectasis in the presence of middle ear underaeration. Atelectatic retraction pockets can lead to the formation of cholesteatomas.

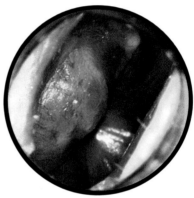

145

145 Acute otitis media with herniation of tympanic membrane, right
As in Fig. **144**, inflammatory exudate under increased pressure has herniated the posterosuperior quadrant of the tympanic membrane laterally. The malleus handle is injected and the middle ear filled with seropurulent exudate. – Atrophic, flaccid areas occur most commonly in the posterosuperior quadrant, Figs **178** and **199**. Since the posterosuperior quadrant of the tympanic membrane herniates laterally more than the other quadrant, the assumption is that such herniation causes dissolution of the fibrous middle layer of this area of the tympanic membrane.

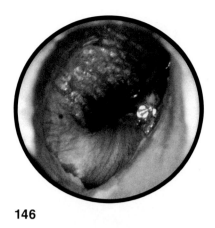

146

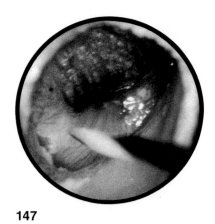

147

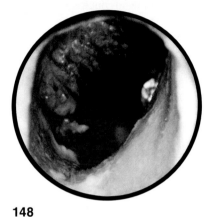

148

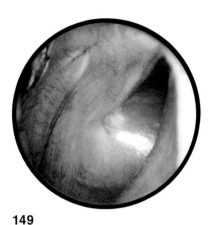

149

146 Acute otitis media with myringotomy and recovery, right

Following an acute upper respiratory infection, this patient suffered a severe earache and fever a few hours before photography of the ear. The tympanic membrane is hyperemic, and the posterior portion bulges laterally. The purulent exudate within the middle ear causes the whitish appearance of the inferior portion of the membrane.

147 Same ear as Figs. 146, 148, and 149

A myringotomy knife is about to perforate the drum.

148 Same ear as Figs. 146, 147, and 149

Immediately following myringotomy, purulent exudate and blood flow into the external auditory canal.

149 Same ear as Figs. 146, 147, and 148

One month following myringotomy and proper antibiotic therapy, the tympanic membrane and middle ear have returned to normal. Acute otitis must be treated and followed by the physician until the ear and hearing have returned to normal.

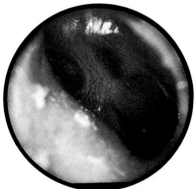

150

150 Acute otitis media, aerotitis, left

This patient took an airplane flight while suffering from an upper respiratory infection. He noted severe earache when the airplane descended. The tympanic membrane is markedly injected and somewhat bulged laterally. There is fluid in the inferior portion of the middle ear which is demonstrated by the arcuate air-fluid interface arching posteriorly from the umbo.

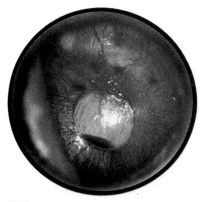

151

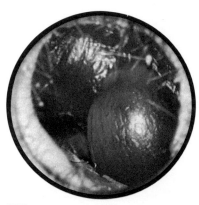

152

151 Acute otitis media, bullous myringitis type, left
There is a small bleb filled with clear serous fluid lying in the center of the pars tensa at the area of the umbo. A little hemorrhagic fluid has settled at the bottom of the bleb.

152 Acute otitis media, bullous myringitis type, left
A large bleb or vesicle occupies the entire posterior half of the tympanic membrane.

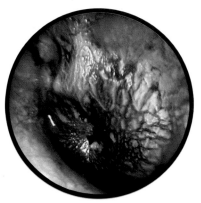

153

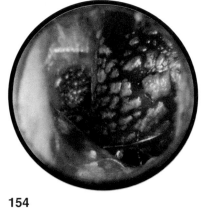

154

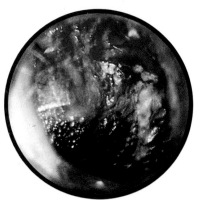

155

153 Acute otitis media, hemorrhagic, grippe type, left
This 31-year-old patient noted sudden onset of earache during an upper respiratory infection. The hemorrhagic involvement of the tympanic membrane extends somewhat onto the adjacent external canal.

154 Acute otitis media, hemorrhagic bullous, grippe type, left
A large hemorrhagic bleb occupies the posterior half of the tympanic membrane and obscures the landmarks.

155 Same ear as Fig. 154, after myringotomy

Mastoiditis

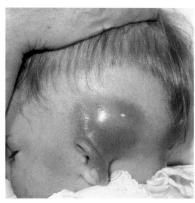

156

156 Acute mastoiditis and subperiosteal abscess, left

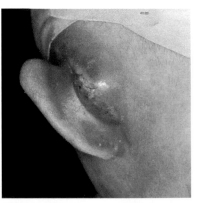

157

157 Recurrent acute mastoiditis with subperiosteal abscess
This 6-year-old child had a simple mastoidectomy two years previously for acute mastoiditis.

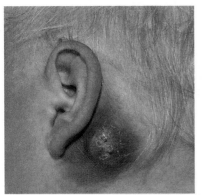

158

158 Abscess in retroauricular lymph node, left
This large abscess in a retroauricular lymph node occurred secondary to a pyogenic infection in the superior retroauricular fold. This lesion must be differentiated from a retroauricular subperiosteal abscess or a Bezold abscess due to an acute mastoiditis. – In this case otoscopy, audiometry, and mastoid x-ray studies were normal. The correct diagnosis was established by finding a primary infected lesion of the scalp in an area drained by the postauricular lymph nodes.

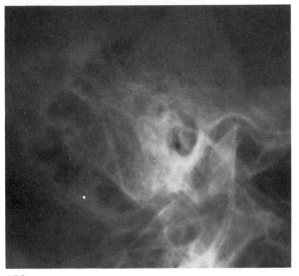

159

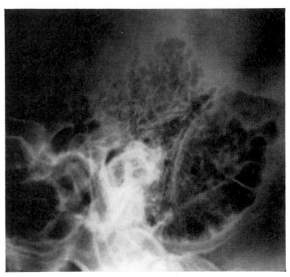

160

159 Acute mastoiditis
Schüller's view of the right mastoid, showing diffuse clouding of the mastoid cells due to loss of air content without evidence of cell wall destruction.

160 Normal mastoid, left
Schüller's view of the normal left mastoid for comparison.

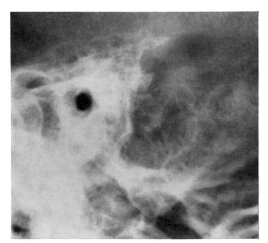

161

161 Suppurative mastoiditis with perisinuous abscess
Law's projection of the left mastoid, showing clouding of the mastoid air cells with some breakdown of the cell walls, partial destruction of the sinus plate.

Chronic Otitis Media

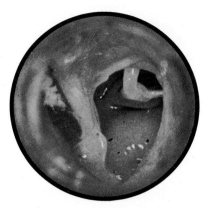

162

162 Chronic otitis media with central perforation, left
There is a large posterior central perforation, and the stapes and incus are seen. The crura and tendon of the stapes can be visualized. There are a few flecks of dark debris on the promontory.

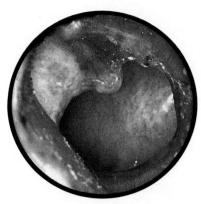

163

163 Chronic otitis media with central perforation, left
A large kidney-shaped perforation occupies both inferior quadrants of the tympanic membrane. The anterosuperior quadrant is thickened by a white tympanosclerotic deposit within the membrane. The promontory mucosa is slightly inflamed.

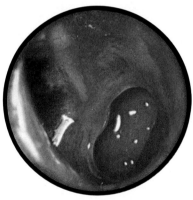

164

164 Chronic otitis media, central perforation with acute recurrent inflammation, left
There is an oval perforation of the posteroinferior pars tensa. The nonperforated tympanic membrane is inflamed and the promontory mucosa is reddened and thickened. The malleus short process and handle are visible.

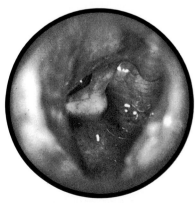

165

165 Chronic otitis media with central perforation, recurrent inflammation, and stapes fixation, right
Only the posterior half of the chronically inflamed middle ear and tympanic membrane are seen due to the narrow external auditory canal. The distal portion of the

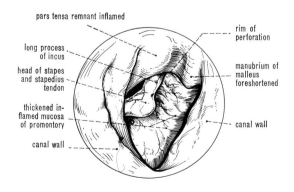

165a

pars tensa remnant inflamed

long process of incus

head of stapes and stapedius tendon

thickened inflamed mucosa of promontory

canal wall

rim of perforation

manubrium of malleus foreshortened

canal wall

manubrium is eroded. The mucosa of the promontory and oval window niche is thickened and inflamed, and there is a seropurulent secretion. The stapes is firmly fixed by the thickened mucosa.

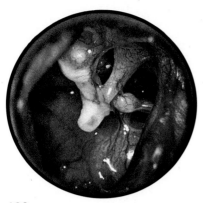

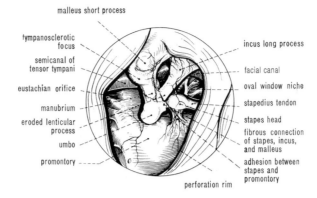

malleus short process

tympanosclerotic focus

semicanal of tensor tympani

eustachian orifice

manubrium

eroded lenticular process

umbo

promontory

incus long process

facial canal

oval window niche

stapedius tendon

stapes head

fibrous connection of stapes, incus, and malleus

adhesion between stapes and promontory

perforation rim

166

166a

166 Chronic otitis media, central perforation, moderate acute recurrent inflammation, left
There is a huge central perforation occupying practically the entire pars tensa. The mucosa of the promontory is inflamed and somewhat thickened. The ossicles are demonstrated in the diagram. There are tympanosclerotic deposits on the manubrium near the short process and on the umbo. The lenticular process has sloughed, and the distal end of the long process of the incus is

adherent to the inferior portion of the manubrium. The posterior margin of the tip of the long process of the incus is still in contact with the head of the stapes. There is a fibrous adhesion between the stapes head and the promontory. The semicanal of the tensor tympani is visible in the anterior superior quadrant. The darkened area immediately below the semicanal is the opening of the eustachian tube into the middle ear.

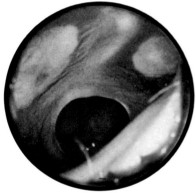

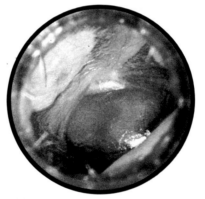

167

168

167 Chronic otitis media with dry central perforation, natural healing, right
There is an inferior, central perforation. There are two white tympanosclerotic plaques in the superior quadrants of the tympanic membrane. The mucosa of the promontory is reddened.

168 Same ear as Fig. 167, following natural healing
Eighteen months later, the perforation has healed with a thin atrophic scar. The rim of the previous perforation is visible.

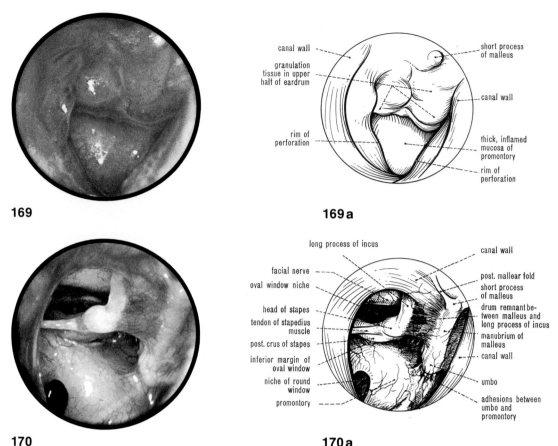

169   **169a**

labels in 169a:
canal wall
granulation tissue in upper half of eardrum
rim of perforation
short process of malleus
canal wall
thick, inflamed mucosa of promontory
rim of perforation

170   **170a**

labels in 170a:
long process of incus
facial nerve
oval window niche
head of stapes
tendon of stapedius muscle
post. crus of stapes
inferior margin of oval window
niche of round window
promontory
canal wall
post. mallear fold
short process of malleus
drum remnant between malleus and long process of incus
manubrium of malleus
canal wall
umbo
adhesions between umbo and promontory

169 Chronic otitis media with central perforation and inflammation, spontaneous subsidence of inflammation, right
Almost the entire pars tensa is perforated, and there is a mass of polypoid granulation tissue involving the malleus handle and the posterosuperior quadrant. The promontory mucosa is thickened and inflamed.

170 Same ear as Fig. 169, seven years later
The chronic inflammation of the ear has resolved spontaneously. The granulation tissue and thick mucosa have receded completely, and now the mucosa of the middle ear appears normal. The structures of the middle ear are identified in the diagram.

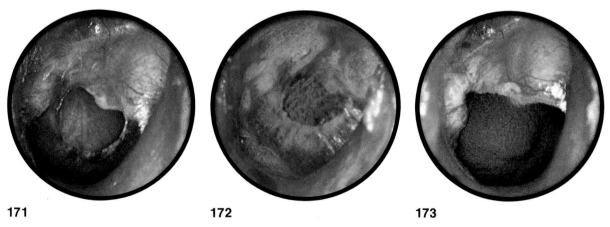

171   **172**   **173**

171 Chronic otitis media, central perforation, right
There is a central perforation inferior to the umbo, occupying about one-fourth of the area of the pars tensa. The perforation has been lightly treated with trichloroacetic acid, visible as a thin, whitish eschar.

172 Same ear as Fig. 171 and 173
Following treatment with trichloroacetic acid, cigarette paper has been placed over the perforation.
173 Same ear as Fig. 171 and 172
Approximately a year after the treatment, the perforation has healed with an atrophic membrane.

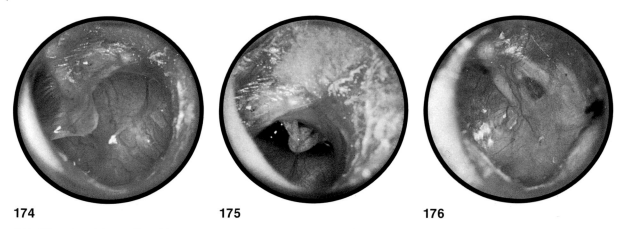

174   **175**   **176**

174 Chronic otitis media with central perforation, before and after vein graft myringoplasty, left

There is a large central perforation involving three-fourths of the tympanic membrane. Only the anterosuperior quadrant remains. The mucosa of the middle ear is normal, and minute adhesive bands extend from the umbo and long process of the incus to the medial wall of the middle ear.

175 Same ear as Figs 174 and 176

The camera is directed posterosuperiorly to show the partially eroded long process of the incus in contact with the head of the stapes. The thin adhesion between the long process of the incus and the head of the stapes with the promontory is clearly seen.

176 Same ear as Figs 174 and 175

One year after a successful vein graft myringoplasty the vein graft is seen as a slightly thickened, pinkish scar occupying the site of the previous perforation.

Sequelae of Chronic Otitis Media, Tympanic Membrane Atrophy, Ossicular Chain Defects

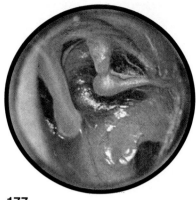

177

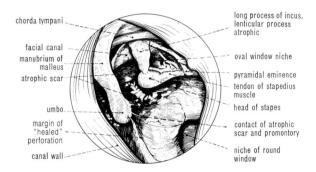

177a

177 Chronic otitis media with retracted, atrophic tympanic membrane, left

The entire posterior half of the tympanic membrane is thin, atrophic, and retracted. The atrophic membrane partially envelops the incus long process, the stapes, and stapedius tendon, and lies in contact with the promon-

tory. The oval and round window niches and the facial nerve are visible through the atrophic scar. There was severe conductive deafness in this ear due to the fixation of the ossicular chain. Although there is no fluid, middle ear aeration is marginal, and there is mild atelectasis of the posterior half of the middle ear.

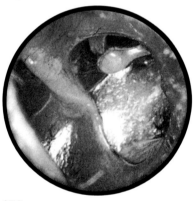

178

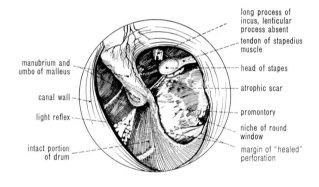

178a

178 Chronic otitis media with atrophic posterior tympanic membrane, left

The posterior half of the tympanic membrane is atrophic and rests on the stapes head and eroded incus long process. The minimal retraction of the atrophic membrane creates a type III tympanoplasty or natural myringostapedioplasty. Middle ear aeration is adequate since the middle ear is air-filled. There is no fluid an only minimal

retraction of the atrophic area. The genesis of atrophic areas in the tympanic membrane is discussed in Figs **143, 144, 145**. Such atrophic areas often thought to be healed perforations, are probably sequelae of herniations and inflammations of the tympanic membrane with destruction of the fibrous layer during prior episodes of acute otitis media.

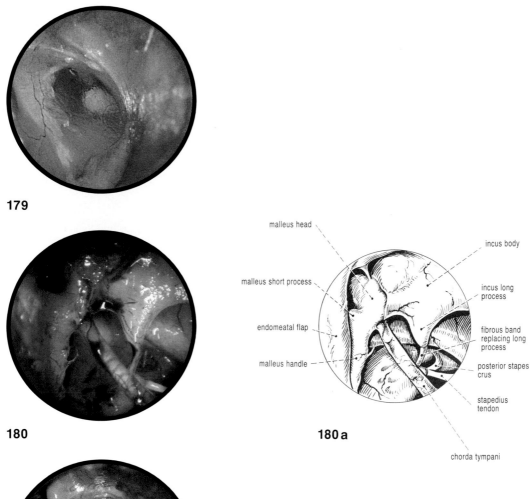

179

180

180a

malleus head

incus body

malleus short process

incus long process

endomeatal flap

fibrous band replacing long process

malleus handle

posterior stapes crus

stapedius tendon

chorda tympani

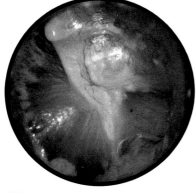

181

179 Chronic otitis media with interrupted ossicular chain, left, same ear as Fig. 181

The posterior superior quadrant of the tympanic membrane is thin and atrophic and lies in the normal plane due to equal pressures of middle and external ears. The head of the stapes appears through the thin atrophic tympanic membrane. There is no contact between the atrophic membrane and the stapes. The long process of the incus is eroded and the ossicular chain is interrupted. This patient had a conductive deafness of approximately 50 decibels due to the interruption of the ossicular chain. The erosion of the long process of the incus probably occurred during an episode of atelectasis in the posterosuperior quadrant which resolved spontaneously. – Figs **196, 199,** and **201** show examples of middle ear atelectasis with skeletonization of the incus and stapes by atrophic areas of the tympanic membrane. An attack of acute otitis during the atelactatic stage could easily result in caries and necrosis of the long process of the incus.

180 Chronic otitis media, eroded long process of incus, surgical findings, left

An endomeatal incision with reflexion of the tympanic membrane and external canal skin anteriorly exposes the replacement of the distal end of the long process of the incus by a thin tenuous core of fibrous tissue. There is conductive deafness since the fibrous core does not conduct sound. – The chorda tympani crosses the stapes head and tendon. The facial nerve passes above the stapes. – The pathology in this ear is similar to that found in Fig. **179**.

181 Chronic otitis media, post incus transposition, same ear as Fig. 179

Following incus transposition between the head of the stapes and the malleus handle, the articular surface of the incus lies in contact with the malleus handle. The superior surface of the incus body protrudes somewhat into the posterosuperior quadrant of the tympanic membrane. The hearing was improved.

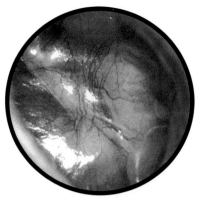

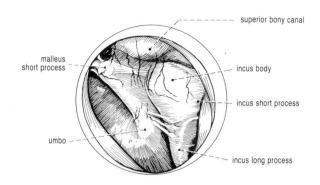

182

182a

182 Chronic otitis media, post incus homograft transposition, left

Following a simple mastoidectomy many years previously, this patient had maximum conductive deafness due to an absent incus. At surgery an incus homograft was transposed between the head of the stapes and the

tympanic membrane. The malleus handle lies to the left, and the transposed body of the incus lies in contact with the posterior superior quadrant of the tympanic membrane over the stapes and oval window area. The long process of the incus extends posteroinferiorly.

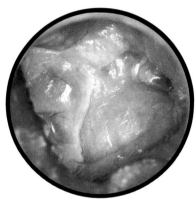

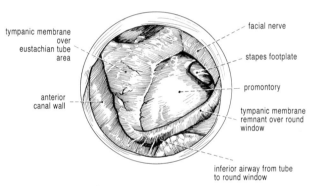

183

183a

183 Chronic otitis media post tympanoplasty Type IV, left

This patient has a functioning Type IV tympanoplasty. The malleus is absent, and the empty oval window and the facial nerve canal lie posterosuperiorly. Inferiorly

the tympanic membrane remnant stretches between the promontory and the anulus laterally to form an enclosed column of air from the aerated anterior eustachian portion of the middle ear to the round window.

Tympanosclerosis

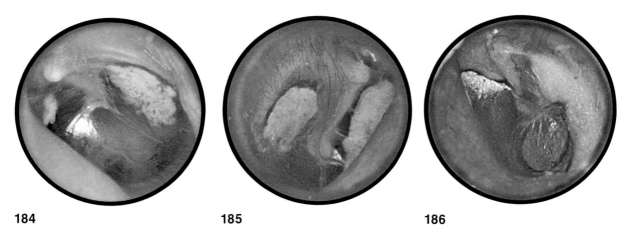

184   **185**   **186**

184 Tympanosclerotic plaques and atrophic tympanic membrane, left
In the superior quadrants there are tympanosclerotic deposits lying within the layers of the tympanic membrane. The inferior quadrants are thin, atrophic, and almost transparent. The atrophic areas move easily with the pneumatic otoscope.

185 Tympanosclerotic plaques, right
There are two rather large tympanosclerotic plaques anterior and posterior to the malleus handle.

186 Tympanosclerotic plaques and atrophic scar, left
There is a large posterior tympanosclerotic plaque and a smaller one anterosuperiorly. Posteroinferiorly an even thinner circular atrophic area probably represents a healed perforation within the larger atrophic area.

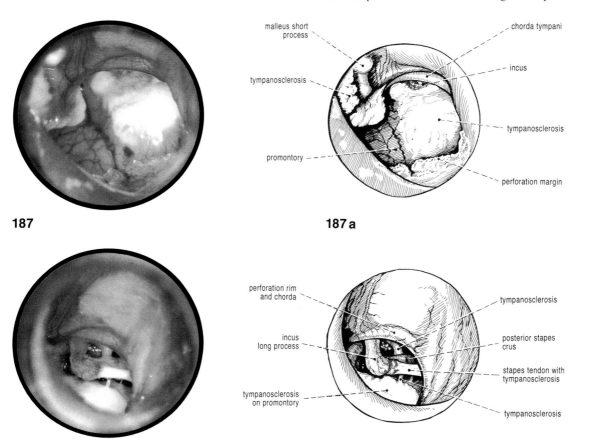

187   **187a**

188   **188a**

187 Tympanosclerosis and perforated tympanic membrane, left
A large central perforation reveals a whitish mass of tympanosclerosis deposited on the promontory. The long process of the incus appears just below the superior margin of the perforation.

188 Same ear as Fig. 187
This is the view of the posterosuperior quadrant of Fig. **187**. Vertical bands of tympanosclerosis fix the stapes to the facial nerve superiorly and to the mass of tympanosclerosis on the promontory inferiorly. There is a deposit of tympanosclerosis on the stapedius muscle tendon.

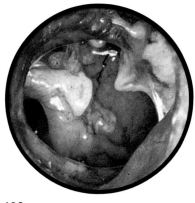

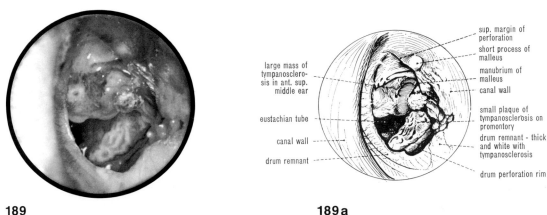

189

189a

189 Tympanosclerosis and perforated tympanic membrane, left

There is a large perforation of the anterior quadrant of the tympanic membrane, and a mass of tympanosclerosis fills this portion of the middle ear. The tym-

panosclerotic mass has the characteristic appearance of whitish, smooth tissue which is firm when palpated. There are deposits of tympanosclerosis on the anterior promontory and the inferior remnant of the tympanic membrane.

190

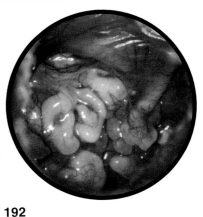

192

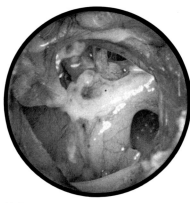

191

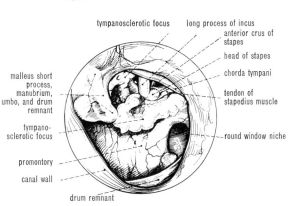

191a

190 Tympanosclerosis with perforated tympanic membrane, right

There is a large central perforation in this ear occupying 75 to 80 percent of the pars tensa. Posterosuperiorly, the long process of the incus articulates with the head of the stapes. On the promontory, just below the oval window niche, is a whitish, rounded tympanosclerotic lesion. The lesion has the typical appearance of tympanosclerosis, described as appearing as if molten wax were dropped onto the promontory and allowed to harden.

191 Tympanosclerosis with perforated tympanic membrane, left, same patient as Fig. 190

The typical whitish, rounded mass of tympanosclerosis extends from the inferior margin of the oval window.

192 Tympanosclerosis with perforated tympanic membrane, right

Multiple small globules of tympanosclerosis on the surface of the promontory appear through a large central perforation. The small globules are firm when palpated.

Atelectasis and Malaeration of the Middle Ear, Chronic Adhesive Otitis Media

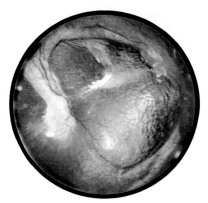

193

193 Chronic otitis media, with atrophic posterior tympanic membrane, left

There is atrophy of almost the entire posterior portion of the tympanic membrane. The remainder of the membrane is normal and has a circular and radial middle fibrous layer. The atrophic membrane is in contact with the slightly eroded long process of the incus and the head of the stapes. The atrophic tympanic membrane lies in the plane of the normal tympanic membrane due to good middle ear aeration and eustachian tube function. The promontory and round window lie opposite the umbo. The demarcation between the atrophic tympanic membrane and the normal anterior tympanic membrane arches inferiorly from the umbo.

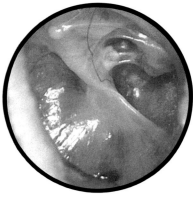

194

194 Middle ear atelectasis, posterior superior quadrant, left

There is atelectasis of the posterior superior quadrant. The atrophic tympanic membrane has partially enveloped the long process of the incus and the head of the stapes. The posterior mallear fold is prominent. A deep fold arches posteriorly from the umbo to demarcate the normal fibrous from the atrophic atelectatic membrane. After continuous middle ear ventilation with a polyethylene tube, the atrophic tympanic membrane returned to the normal, anular plane.

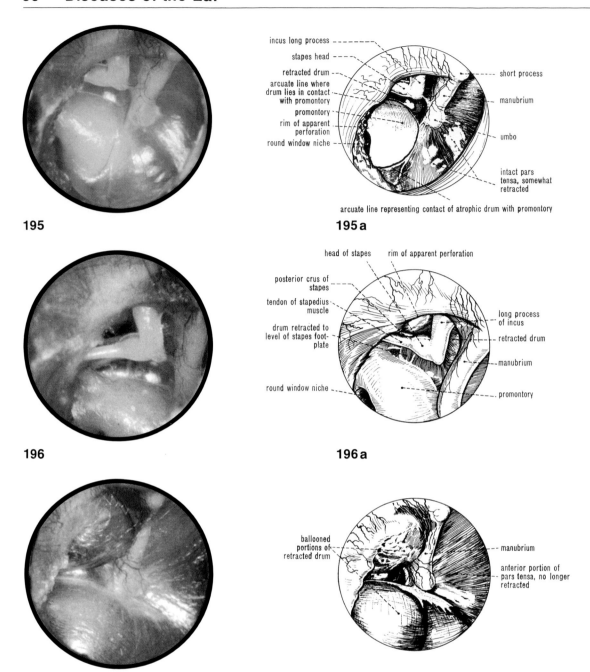

195

incus long process
stapes head
retracted drum
arcuate line where
drum lies in contact
with promontory
promontory
rim of apparent
perforation
round window niche

short process
manubrium
umbo
intact pars
tensa, somewhat
retracted

arcuate line representing contact of atrophic drum with promontory

195 a

196

head of stapes   rim of apparent perforation
posterior crus of
stapes
tendon of stapedius
muscle
drum retracted to
level of stapes foot-
plate
round window niche

long process
of incus
retracted drum
manubrium
promontory

196 a

197

ballooned
portions of
retracted drum

manubrium
anterior portion of
pars tensa, no longer
retracted

197 a

195 Middle ear atelectasis, right
The posterior portion of the middle ear is atelectatic, and the retracted, atrophic membrane lies on the promontory, round window niche, stapes and incus long process. There is no fluid in the middle ear.

196 Same ear as Figs 195, 197, and 198
When directed superiorly, the camera shows the partial envelopment of the incus long process, stapes, and stapes tendon by the atrophic, tympanic membrane. A fold of the atrophic membrane is draped over the stapes to the promontory.

197 Same ear as Figs 195, 196, and 198 after politzerization
After politzerization, the atelectatic nature of the mid-

dle ear is apparent. The atrophic membrane has ballooned laterally. Ballooning of the atrophic membrane indicates preservation of the potential space between the medial surface of the collapsed membrane and the mucosa of the medial wall of the middle ear. The normal, fibrous anterior tympanic membrane is minimally expanded.

198 Same ear as Figs 195, 196, and 197 after middle ear aeration with an indwelling polyethylene tube
Following prolonged middle ear aeration, the atrophic membrane has contracted and shifted laterally to the normal plane of the tympanic membrane. The stapes and incus long process are no longer enveloped by the atrophic membrane.

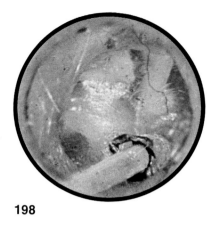

198

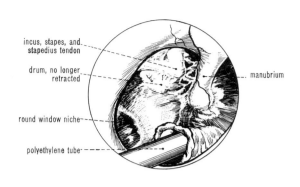

incus, stapes, and
stapedius tendon

drum, no longer
retracted

round window niche

polyethylene tube

manubrium

198 a

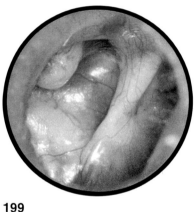

199

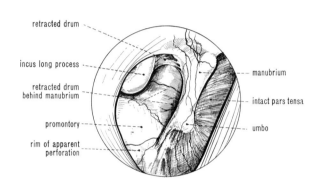

retracted drum

incus long process

retracted drum
behind manubrium

promontory

rim of apparent
perforation

manubrium

intact pars tensa

umbo

199 a

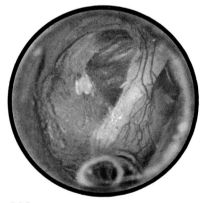

200

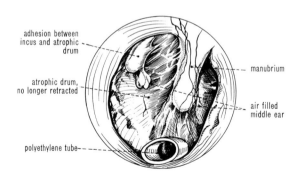

adhesion between
incus and atrophic
drum

atrophic drum,
no longer retracted

polyethylene tube

manubrium

air filled
middle ear

200 a

199 Middle ear atelectasis, right

The entire posterior half of the middle ear is atelectatic and the tympanic membrane is so deeply retracted that the membrane appears perforated. The atrophic membrane has enveloped the long process of the incus and the stapes head. The yellow-brown color of the tympanic membrane is due to serous fluid within the middle ear. The anterior portion of the tympanic membrane is not atelectatic because of persistence of the fibrous middle layer.

200 Same ear as Fig. 199 following middle ear ventilation

After middle ear ventilation with an indwelling tube, the atelectasis is relieved, and the atrophic membrane has "deretracted" and contracted to the normal plane. There is a persistent adhesion between the atrophic membrane and long process of the incus, and the middle ear is air-filled and has a normal pearl gray color.

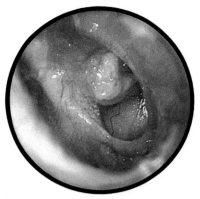

201

201 Middle ear atelectasis, left
There is severe atelectasis of the posterior portion of the
left middle ear. The remaining ear space is filled with
yellowish fluid. The atrophic tympanic membrane has
enveloped and skeletonized the incus long process and
stapes. Medially the membrane lies in contact with the
promontory.

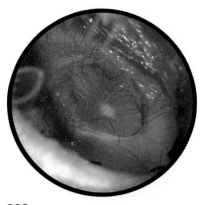

202

**202 Same ear as in Fig. 201 after prolonged middle ear
        aeration with an indwelling polyethylene tube**
The thin posterosuperior quadrant of the tympanic
membrane has contracted and migrated laterally to the
normal anular plane. The membrane has "disenveloped" itself from the long process of the incus and from
the stapes.

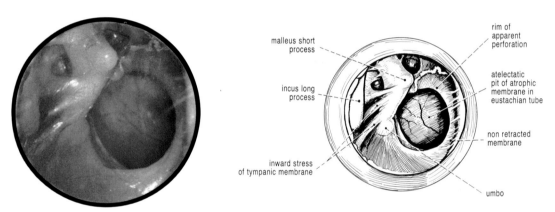

203

**203 Middle ear atelectasis, anterosuperior quadrant,
        post intubation, right**
There is a severe, deep atelectatic pocket in the anterior
superior quadrant of the right middle ear. The remaining
portion of the middle ear is filled with serous fluid which
gives the tympanic membrane a dark yellow cast. The
atrophic and ectatic anterosuperior tympanic membrane
lies in contact with the medial wall of the middle ear and
has been forced by negative pressure into the eustachian
tube portion of the middle ear. The short process of the
malleus is prominent, and the posterior superior quadrant of the tympanic membrane, which contains a circular and radiating fibrous middle layer, is retracted and
stressed medially. The long process of the incus is just

203 a

visible at the posterior margin of the photograph. To enlarge and retract so deeply, the thin atrophic area of the
tympanic membrane increases its surface area under the
trophic influences of negative middle ear pressure. Severely atelectatic ears such as this, unless studied carefully under the operating microscope, can be mistaken
for chronic otitis with a perforated tympanic membrane.
– Six years previously, this patient had a myringotomy
and polyethylene tube insertion in the anterosuperior
quadrant. The tube extruded spontaneously and the patient did not return for four years. The polyethylene tube
destroyed the middle fibrous layer of the anterosuperior
quadrant, and recurrent middle ear malaeration produced the atelectasis.

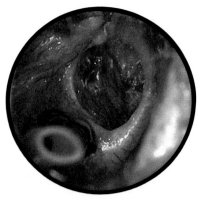

204

204 Same ear as Figs 203 and 205 immediately after insertion af a polyethylene tube
There is a polyethylene tube in the posteroinferior portion of the tympanic membrane. With a small aspirating tube, a portion of the atrophic tympanic membrane was aspirated laterally and appears as the reddened membrane in the anterosuperior quadrant. The negative pressure in the ear was so great that the retracted, tympanic membrane could not be elevated from the promontory and eustachian tube area until the vacuum was relieved with the polyethylene tube airvent.

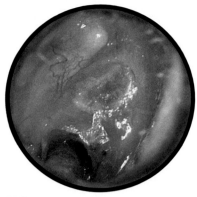

205

205 Same ear as Figs 203 and 204 two months after middle ear ventilation with a polyethylene tube
The atelectasis of the middle ear has been relieved, and the atrophic membrane has contracted and migrated to the plane of the normal tympanic membrane. The polyethylene tube lies inferiorly.

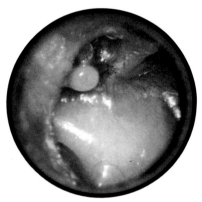

206

206 Middle ear atelectasis, right
Almost the entire middle ear of this ten-year-old child is markedly atelectatic. The atrophic tympanic membrane lies in contact with the promontory and envelops the head of the stapes and the long process of the incus. The atrophic membrane is applied to the round window niche posteroinferiorly. The malleus handle lies anterosuperiorly.

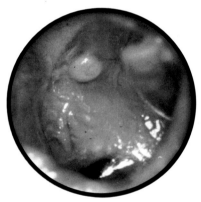

207

207 Same ear as Fig. 206, after middle ear ventilation with a polyethylene tube
Several months following correction of the atelectasis by continuous middle ear aeration with a polyethylene tube, the atrophic membrane has come away from the promontory and is close to the normal anular plane of the tympanic membrane. The atrophic membrane still lies in contact with the head of the stapes but has "disenveloped" itself from the long process of the incus and the crura of the stapes. The membrane has also shifted laterally away from the round and oval windows. The polyethylene tube lies anteriorly.

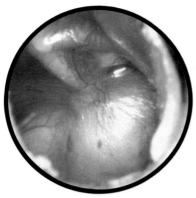

208

208 Middle ear atelectasis, severe, left
The thin, atrophic, retracted tympanic membrane has come to lie on the promontory inferiorly and in contact with the long process of the incus posterosuperiorly. Anterosuperiorly, a portion of the tympanic membrane with a fibrous layer resists the negative middle ear pressure and lies in the normal position. Accompanying serous fluid casts an overall yellow color to the tympanic membrane.

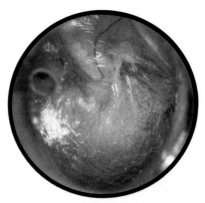

209

209 Same ear as Fig. 208 one year after continuous middle ear aeration
The polyethylene tube lies in the anterosuperior quadrant. The atelectasis is relieved, and the tympanic membrane has come away from the promontory to lie in the plane of the normal tympanic membrane. The serous fluid is gone. The tympanic membrane appears gray, semitranslucent, and has an almost normal appearance.

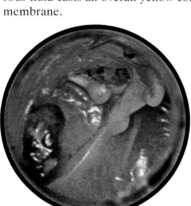

210

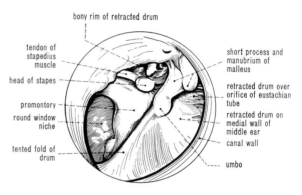

bony rim of retracted drum

tendon of stapedius muscle

head of stapes

promontory

round window niche

tented fold of drum

short process and manubrium of malleus

retracted drum over orifice of eustachian tube

retracted drum on medial wall of middle ear

canal wall

umbo

210a

210 Chronic adhesive otitis media with irreversible atelectasis, right
The middle ear is atelectatic and the atrophic tympanic membrane lies on the medial wall of the middle ear. The atrophic membrane is draped over the stapes and stapes tendon. The membrane is deeply retracted into the round window niche posteriorly and onto the medial wall of the middle ear anteriorly. – Middle ear ventilation in this ear failed to re-expand the middle ear because of obliteration of the potential space between the medial surface of the atrophic membrane and the structures of the medial wall of the middle ear.

Cholesteatomas of the Middle Ear and Mastoid
Pathogenesis of Cholesteatoma from Middle Ear Atelectasis

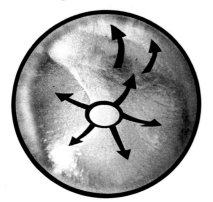

211

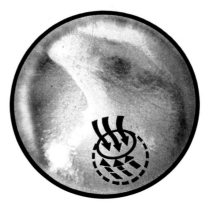

212

211 Migration of superficial epithelium, left
This composite demonstrates the centrifugal migration of the cornified layer of the epithelium of the suface of the tympanic membrane. The migration begins at the umbo and spreads centrifugally through 360°.

212 Migration of epithelial debris into mesotympanic atelectatic pocket, left
This composite diagram illustrates how the superficial cornified epithelium of the tympanic membrane migrates centrifugally from the umbo into the depths of an atelectatic pocket in the inferior portion of the middle ear. In a deep pocket, the cornified epithelium cannot migrate out of the atelectatic pocket and a cholesteatoma forms.

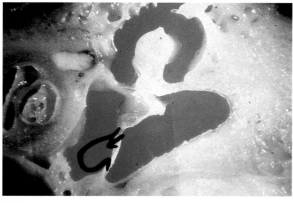

213

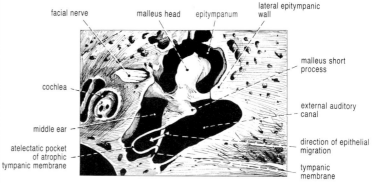

213a

213 Migration of epithelium into atelectatic pocket, left
This diagram illustrates the migration of superficial cornified epithelium into an atelectatic pocket. The dia-

gram is superimposed on a coronal cross section of a temporal bone at the level of the external auditory canal, the malleus, the facial nerve and the cochlea.

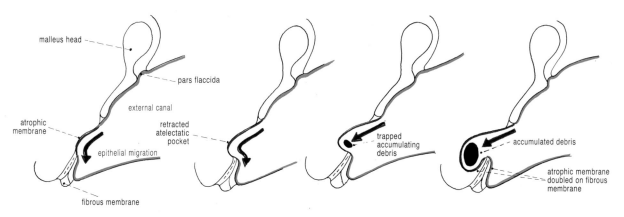

214 a   **b**   **c**   **d**

214 Genesis of cholesteatoma in an atelectic pocket
These diagrams illustrate migration of cornified epithelial cells on the surface of the tympanic membrane in various stages of atelectasis and cholesteatoma development.
a) Negative middle ear pressure causes slight retraction of an atrophic portion of the tympanic membrane. This shallow pit permits easy migration of epithelium peripherally.
b) With increased negative middle ear pressure, the pit deepens, but still permits peripheral migration.
c) In a deeper pit, cornified epithelial debris begins to be trapped medial to the rigid peripheral remnant of the tympanic membrane. The peripheral membrane is resistant to negative pressure within the middle ear be-

cause of the presence of circular and radiating fibers within the membrane segment.
d) In a still deeper pit the cornified epithelial debris is unable to surmount the sharp edge of the rigid peripheral tympanic membrane segment. Epithelial debris, denied egress, accumulates within the pit, causing enlargement and stretching of the atrophic tympanic membrane which surrounds it. The atrophic membrane doubles itself on the medial surface of the peripheral, rigid tympanic membrane segment. Further accumulation of debris enlarges the pit and leads to encystment and cholesteatoma formation.

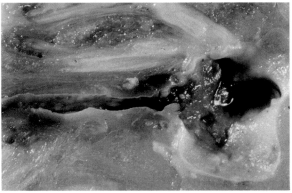

215

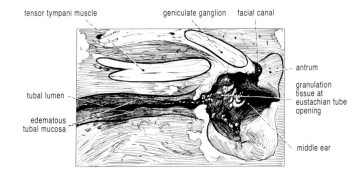

215a

215 Eustachian tube stenosis and cholesteatoma, temporal bone cross section, Stenvers plane, right
There is an extensive cholesteatoma of the middle ear and mastoid in this temporal bone cross section cut at the level of the mastoid process, the middle ear, and the eustachian tube. The Stenvers plane bisects the eustachian tube. The mucosa of the eustachian tube is markedly thickened from the middle ear orifice to the cartilaginous portion, and the tubal lumen is stenosed. There is

granulation tissue on the anterior wall at the ostium of the eustachian tube. The smooth, middle ear cavity is lined with cholesteatoma matrix which extends posterosuperiorly into the mastoid. The stapes superstructure is absent, and the stapes footplate lies in the oval window under the facial nerve. Compare these findings with the normal eustachian tube at the same level in Figs **92–95**.

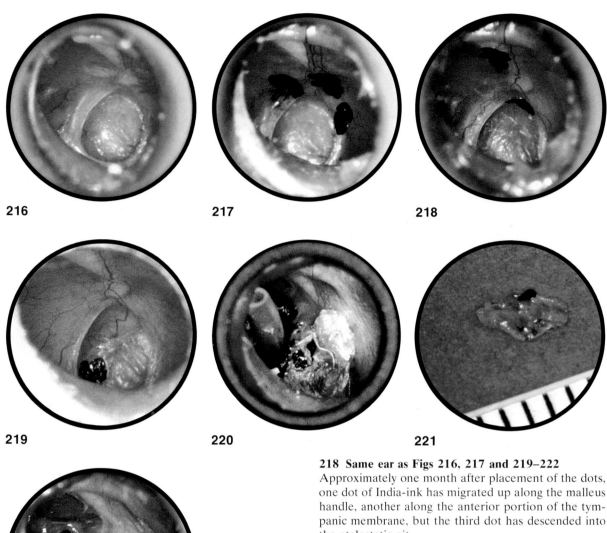

216   217   218

219   220   221

222

216 Middle ear atelectasis, demonstration of migration of epithelial debris to form incipient cholesteatoma, left

The clinical significance of Figs **211–215** is demonstrated in this series of photographs. Figs **216–222** are serial photographs of the ear of a child with a small atelectatic pocket in the inferior portion of the tympanic membrane. – In Fig. **216** the entire tympanic membrane has a yellowish-blue color due to serous fluid which fills the middle ear. This series of photographs shows epithelial migration into the pocket and accumulation of epithelial debris to form an incipient cholesteatoma.

217 Same ear as Figs 216 and 218–222

Three India-ink dots were placed at the margin of the atelectatic pocket to demonstrate the migration of the desquamated stratified epithelium peripherally from the center of the tympanic membrane.

218 Same ear as Figs 216, 217 and 219–222

Approximately one month after placement of the dots, one dot of India-ink has migrated up along the malleus handle, another along the anterior portion of the tympanic membrane, but the third dot has descended into the atelectatic pit.

219 Same ear as Figs 216–218 and 220–222

One month later, there is further migration of the India-ink dot into the depths of the pit inferiorly. Epithelial debris is beginning to accumulate and fill the atelectatic pit.

220 Same ear as Figs 216–219 and 221, 222

A polyethylene tube has been inserted and the atelectatic pit partially everted. The small nidus of epithelial debris from within the atelectatic pit and early cholesteatoma now lies on the surface of the tympanic membrane in the plane of the normal tympanic membrane. The atelectatic pit is shrinking and migrating laterally.

221 Same ear as Figs 216–220 and 222

This is the epithelial nidus seen in Fig. **220** after removal from the surface of the tympanic membrane. The nidus contains the India-ink dot seen in Fig. **218**.

222 Same ear as Figs 216–221

One month after an indwelling polyethylene tube was placed in the middle ear and the nidus removed, the atelectatic area has contracted and lies in the plane of the normal tympanic membrane. The middle ear is filled with air and there is a normal grayish color of the tympanic membrane.

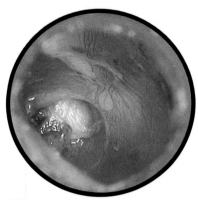

223

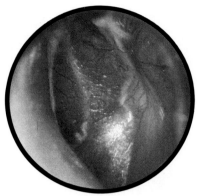

224

223 Atelectasis of the middle ear with a developing cholesteatoma, left

Figs **223** and **224** demonstrate the dilemma associated with the use of middle ear tubes. There is a deep retracted atelectatic pocket filled with a nidus of desquamated epithelial debris formed from entrapped epithelial debris from the surface of the atelectatic pit. At this time the patient was seven years old. The middle ear appears air-filled. Because of serous otitis media two years previously, a polyethylene tube was inserted in the anterosuperior quadrant at the site of the atelectatic pocket. The tube extruded leaving a thin atrophic tympanic membrane, and the middle ear became atelectatic with recurrent malaeration of the middle ear. Epithelial debris accumulated within the atelectatic pocket as seen in Figs **216–222**.

224 Same ear as Fig. 223, five years later

The atelectatic pocket filled with epithelial debris in Fig. **223** was everted and evacuated, and a polyethylene tube was reinserted in the anterosuperior quadrant. This resulted in resolution of the retracted atelectatic pocket. In the ensuing five years the tube extruded but middle ear aeration became normal as the patient matured. The middle ear is air-filled, and the retracted atrophic membrane is re-expanded to lie in the plane of the normal tympanic membrane. The atrophic area of the tympanic membrane lies anteriorly at the margin of the external auditory canal.

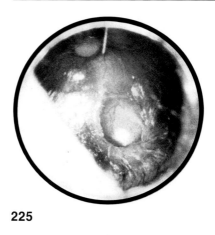

225

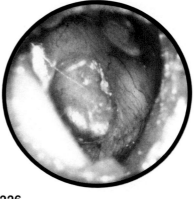

226

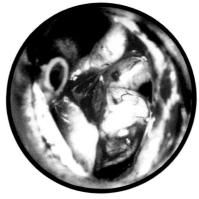

227

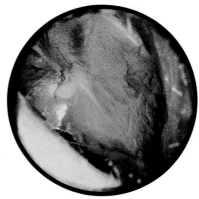

228

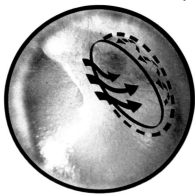

229

225 Middle ear cholesteatoma, treatment by eversion and ventilation, left

The middle ear of a five-year-old child is filled with a yellow-brownish serous fluid. Below the umbo, which lies superiorly, there is a small retracted atelectatic pit which appears to be a small perforation. Microscopic otoscopy revealed the lesion to be an atelectatic pit and not a perforation.

226 Same ear as in Figs 225, 227, and 228, approximately one year later

The interior atelectatic retraction pit has now enlarged and is filled with a nidus of epithelial debris to form a cholesteatoma. The cholesteatoma is visible as a whitish mass in the posteroinferior portion of the mesotympanum beneath the overlying intact tympanic membrane. Above the cholesteatoma cyst is a small air bubble showing the presence of the middle ear fluid. The patient failed to return for scheduled visits in the year-long interval between Figs **226** and **225**.

227 Same ear as Figs 225, 226, and 228

Following an inferior tympanotomy, the skin of the posterior canal wall is dissected and reflected anteriorly, and the whitish cyst lies in the middle ear just below the promontory and round window niche. The cyst was everted and the epithelial debris evacuated. A polyethylene tube was inserted anterosuperiorly.

228 Same ear as Figs 225–227

One year after surgery, the indwelling polyethylene tube lies inferiorly, and the retracted atelectatic pit is no longer present. The atrophic area below the umbo in the normal plane represents the site from which the atelectatic area developed and filled with debris to form the small cholesteatoma of Fig. **226**. The middle ear is air-filled. See Figs **214** and **216–222**.

229 Migration of epithelial debris into posterosuperior atelectatic pocket, left

This composite shows one method of pathogenesis of posterosuperior cholesteatomas. Superficial cornified epithelial debris migrates centrifugally from the umbo and the area posterior to the malleus handle into the depths of a posterosuperior atelectatic pocket. The atelectatic pocket forms from an atrophic area of the tympanic membrane due to negative middle ear pressure. See Figs **144, 145, 199,** and **201**. – Migration of epithelial debris out of the atelectatic pit is prevented by accumulation of the debris medial and posterosuperior to the posterosuperior bony external canal wall.

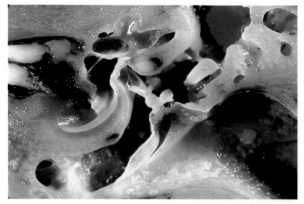

230

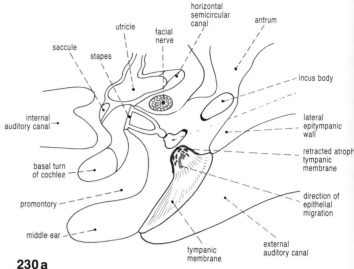

230 a

230 Cholesteatoma genesis from the posterosuperior pars tensa, frontal cross section at level of stapes and long process of incus, left

These diagrams show the pathogenesis of some cholesteatomas of the pars tensa.

230 a There is minimal atelectasis of the posterosuperior portion of the middle ear. A small atrophic area of the pars tensa of the tympanic membrane lies in contact with the lenticular process of the incus. The long process of the incus is missing between the incus body lying in the epitympanum and the lenticular process. The arrow indicates the direction of the migration of the superficial layer of the epithelium of the tympanic membrane. Epithelial debris migrates easily out of the shallow atelectatic pit.

230 b Continued negative middle ear pressure exerts a trophic effect on the thin atrophic area of the pars tensa. The total surface of the atrophic area increases and retracts deeper and deeper into the middle ear and epitympanum. Cholesteatomas originating from atrophic areas of the pars tensa generally tend to infiltrate into the antrum medial to the ossicles, eroding the long process of the incus as they enlarge. – The arrow shows the migratory course of the superficial epithelium. Epithelial debris tends to be caught and to collect in the deeper, narrower reaches of the atelectatic pockets. The lenticular process is eroded.

230 c In this stage of the genesis of cholesteatoma, there is a nidus of epithelial debris which has accumulated in the depths of the atelectatic pocket. Continued desquamation from the inner walls of the atelectatic pocket cause enlargement and encystment in the epitympanum and aditus. In this diagram, the early cholesteatoma has extended to the aditus medial to the incus. The incus is partially eroded and displaced laterally. – The arrow shows direction of migration of epithelium and epithelial debris which adds to the mass of epithelial debris within the lumen of the sac.

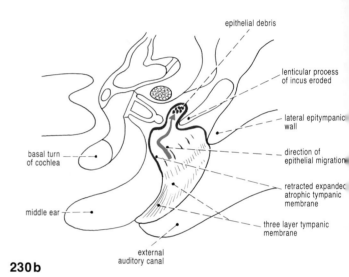

230 b

230 c

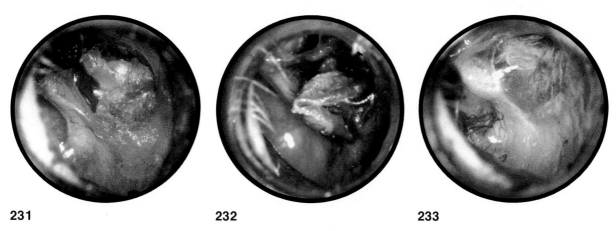

231   **232**   **233**

231 Disencystment of an early cholesteatoma of the posterosuperior portion of the pars tensa, left
There is a deep atelectatic pocket in the posterior portion of the left ear with a crust of necrotic epithelial debris filling the lumen of the pocket. The thin atrophic, atelectatic membrane partially envelops the long process of the incus and the head of the stapes.

232 Same ear as Figs 231 and 233
The necrotic epithelial nidus has been removed, and the cholesteatoma sac everted.

233 Same ear as Figs 231 and 232
Six weeks after continuous middle ear ventilation with a polyethylene tube, the atelectatic pocket has disappeared, having shrunk and migrated laterally.

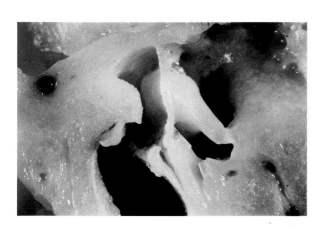

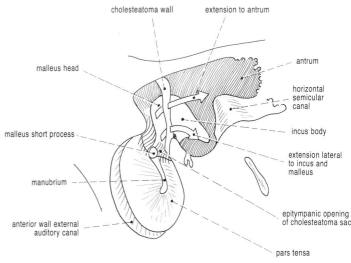

234 Cholesteatoma genesis from pars flaccida, sagittal cross section of epitympanic cholesteatoma, left
There is a small epitympanic cholesteatoma in this cross section which is at the level of the opening of the sac. The pars tensa lies medially and is not visible in the photograph. The cholesteatoma sac originates from the pars flaccida and extends superiorly to the tegmen of the epitympanum. The posterior wall of the sac extends laterally from the body of the incus. The medial sac wall lies on the head of the malleus, and the anterior wall is applied to the anterior epitympanic wall. – This lesion has evacuated itself spontaneously and, since no epithelial debris has accumulated in the sac, the sac has not enlarged. The posterior half of the epitympanum and the antrum are uninvolved. – The arrows in the illustration show the direction of expansion and extension of epitympanic cholesteatomas, lateral to the ossicles into the antrum and mastoid.

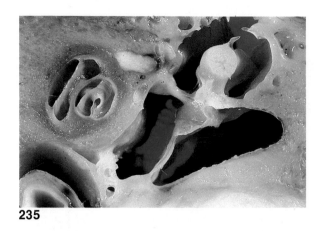

235

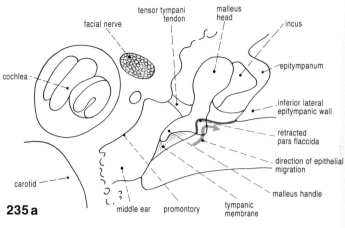

235 a

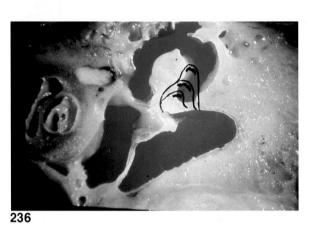

236

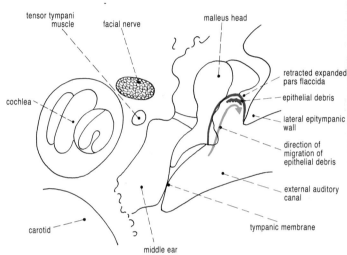

236 a

235 Cholesteatoma genesis from the pars flaccida, coronal cross section at the level of the malleus head

These illustrations show the pathogenesis of epitympanic cholesteatomas from pars flaccida retractions and attic atelectasis. – The pars flaccida is retracted just above the short process of the malleus. The arrow indicates the migratory course of the epithelium of the surface of the tympanic membrane. Such a shallow epitympanic pit does not interfere with migration.

236 Cholesteatoma genesis, coronal cross section, progression from Fig. 235

Continued negative middle ear pressure exerts a trophic effect, increases the surface area of the pars flaccida and allows deeper retraction and enlargement of the intact pars flaccida membrane. – The arrow shows the direction of migration of superficial epithelium. A nidus of epithelial debris becomes trapped and accumulates in the depth of the atelectatic epitympanic pocket. – Erosion of the inferior margin of the lateral epitympanic wall is beginning. – Cholesteatomas arising from the pars flaccida enlarge and reach the epitympanum generally lateral to the ossicles. – Further accumulation of desquamated epithelial debris in the depths of the atelectatic pars flaccida pouch causes encystment, and an early cholesteatom forms. – Epitympanic cholesteatomas expand with further desquamation of epithelial debris from the luminal surface of the sac. Erosion of the bony lateral wall of the epitympanum and medial displacement of the ossicles occur.

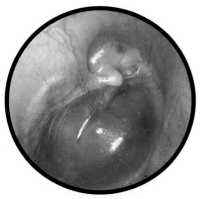

237

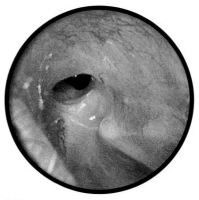

238

237 Pars flaccida retraction with secretory otitis media, right

The middle ear is filled with serous fluid and the pars flaccida deeply retracted due to middle ear malaeration. Retractions as illustrated here and in the preceding illustrations demonstrate the pathogenesis of epitympanic cholesteatomas.

238 Cholesteatoma, early epitympanic, pars flaccida, left

There is an apparent deep epitympanic perforation in

the pars flaccida anterosuperior to the malleus short process. There is no inflammation or accumulated epithelial debris visible. In reality this is not a perforation of the pars flaccida but the opening of a blind retraction sac which extends into the epitympanum for a short distance. – The sac in the epitympanum is probably of the same extent as the lesion in Fig. **236**. – Tomography in an ear such as this will reveal whether the lesion is a shallow pit, or whether there is extension into the epitympanum and antrum.

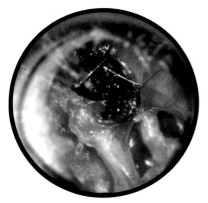

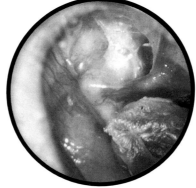

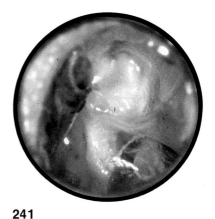

239   **240**   **241**

239 Pathogenesis of cholesteatoma of the pars flaccida, disencystment with ventilation, left

A large crust has eroded the notch of Rivinus. The crust consists of black necrotic epithelial debris and is the nidus of a small cholesteatoma of the pars flaccida.

240 Same ear as Figs 239 and 241

After topical steroid antibiotic therapy, the necrotic cholesteatoma nidus was removed from the retracted but intact pars flaccida to reveal an enlarged notch of Rivinus above the short process of the malleus. The posterior mallear fold is prominent, and the everted atelectatic sac of the posterior superior quadrant is seen posteriorly and inferiorly. This is the same ear as Fig. **231**. – We found combined cholesteatomas arising from both the pars tensa and pars flaccida in one-fourth of the affected ears we studied.

241 Same ear as Figs 239 and 240

After six weeks of continuous indwelling polyethylene tube middle ear ventilation, the retracted pars flaccida has contracted to the normal position and the epitympanic atelectasis is relieved. The polyethylene tube lies to the left. The neck and head of the malleus are seen above the short process of the malleus. The retracted membrane, which extended into the attic posteriorly, now lies stretched between the margin of the notch of Rivinus and the neck of the malleus. The entire pars flaccida is intact and there are no retracted areas. The retracted sac of the pars tensa has also returned to the anular plane.

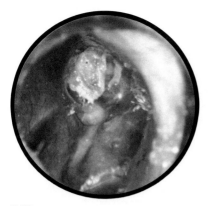

242

242 Early pars flaccida cholesteatoma, disencystment, removal of epithelial nidus, and middle ear ventilation, right

Before photography only a small crust was visible in the pars flaccida area. The crust was grasped with a micro hook and the nidus of the epithelial debris was extracted from the epitympanum. The ectatic pars flaccida has been everted and extends inferiorly from the somewhat enlarged notch of Rivinus.

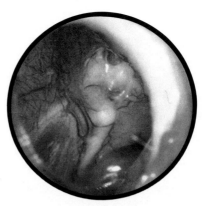

243

243 Same ear as Fig. 242

Following prolonged middle ear ventilation with an indwelling polyethylene tube, the retracted pars flaccida has now contracted and migrated externally into the eroded notch of Rivinus. A portion of the neck and head of the malleus are seen, and the pars flaccida, no longer retracted, extends from the anterior portion of the neck of the malleus to the anterior margin of the notch of Rivinus. The anterior mallear ligament is visible through the eroded notch of Rivinus.

Pars Tensa, Acquired Cholesteatomas

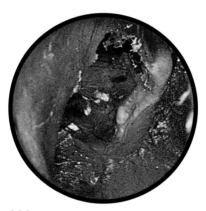

244

244 Cholesteatoma pars tensa, right

There is a large posterosuperior marginal type of perforation with erosion of the medial portion of the posterosuperior bony canal wall at the sulcus tympanicus. The facial nerve appears on the medial wall of the middle ear. There is a small amount of necrotic epithelial debris at the superior margin of the perforation. – As in pars flaccida lesions, the perforation is actually the mouth of an epidermoid cyst. Pars tensa cholesteatomas usually extend into the mastoid antrum and epitympanum medial to the ossicular chain.

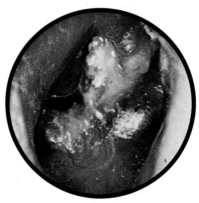

245

245 Same ear as Fig. 244, two years later

In two years the lesion has enlarged and become inflamed. Necrotic epithelial debris fills the lumen of the perforation, and there is a granuloma at the posterosuperior margin of the perforation. At surgery there was a large cholesteatoma filling the epitympanum and antrum with a fistula in the horizontal semicircular canal.

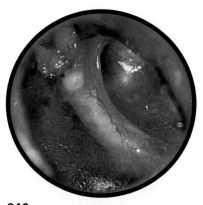

246

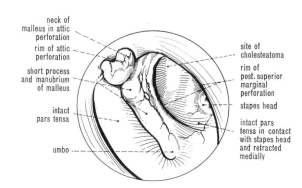

246 a

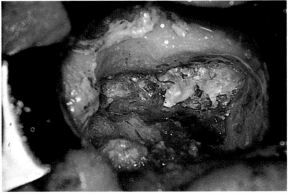

247

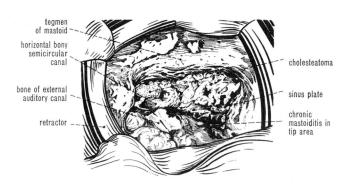

247 a

246 Cholesteatoma, pars tensa, left

There is a posterosuperior marginal perforation which appears to be free of discharge. The posterosuperior bony canal wall is slightly eroded. There is also a small pars flaccida perforation with minimal erosion of the notch of Rivinus. Approximately 25 percent of cholesteatomas occur with combined perforations of the pars flaccida and pars tensa similar to the lesion in this ear.

247 Same ear as Fig. 246, surgical pathology

At surgery an extensive cholesteatoma involved the epitympanum, antrum and mastoid process. Necrotic epithelial debris fills the lumen of the cholesteatoma.

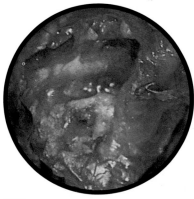

248

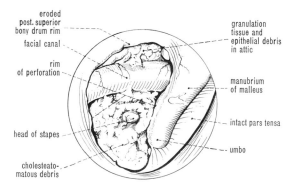

248 a

248 Cholesteatoma, pars tensa, right

There is a large posterosuperior marginal perforation with erosion of the posterosuperior bony canal wall. The lumen of the perforation is filled with necrotic epithelial

debris. There is granulation tissue in the superior part of the perforation. The facial nerve and stapes head partially covered by epithelial debris are visible on the medial wall of the middle ear.

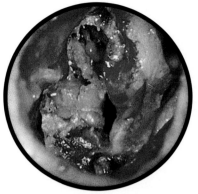

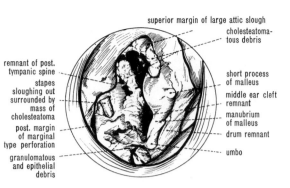

superior margin of large attic slough

cholesteatoma-tous debris

remnant of post. tympanic spine

short process of malleus

stapes sloughing out surrounded by mass of cholesteatoma

middle ear cleft remnant

manubrium of malleus

post. margin of marginal type perforation

drum remnant

umbo

granulomatous and epithelial debris

249

249a

249 Cholesteatoma, pars tensa, extensive, right
There is a large perforation of the posterior portion of the pars tensa and erosion of the posterosuperior bony canal wall reaching into the epitympanum. The middle

ear is filled with necrotic epithelial debris and granulation tissue. The necrotic stapes crura and head have been sloughed from the footplate and lie posterosuperiorly within the mass of epithelial debris.

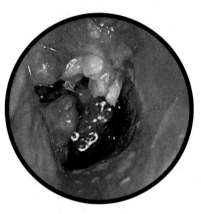

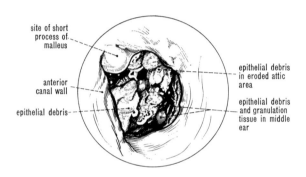

site of short process of malleus

epithelial debris in eroded attic area

anterior canal wall

epithelial debris and granulation tissue in middle ear

epithelial debris

250

250a

250 Cholesteatoma, pars tensa extensive, left
There is a total absence of the tympanic membrane. There is a small granuloma over the short process of the malleus, and the middle ear is filled with necrotic

epithelial debris and granulation tissue. The posterosuperior bony canal wall and the lateral attic wall are eroded.

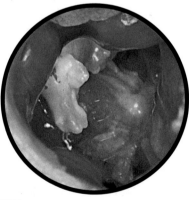

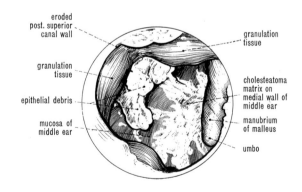

eroded post. superior canal wall

granulation tissue

granulation tissue

epithelial debris

cholesteatoma matrix on medial wall of middle ear

mucosa of middle ear

manubrium of malleus

umbo

251

251a

251 Cholesteatoma, pars tensa, extensive, right
The posterior portion of the tympanic membrane is absent, and the middle ear is filled with granulation tissue and necrotic epithelial debris. The necrotic epithelial

debris sheds into the posterosuperior portion of the middle ear from a large mastoid and epitympanic cholesteatoma. The malleus handle is covered with granulation tissue and lies at the right of the photograph.

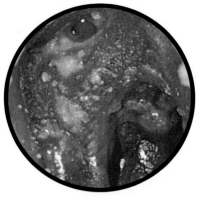

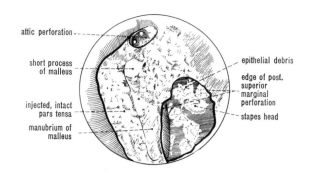

252

252a

252 Cholesteatoma, pars tensa and pars flaccida with acute exacerbation, left

This patient had a long history of chronic ear discharge and hearing loss with recent onset of acute, severe earache, temporal headache, increased discharge and fever. – Intracranial complications most often occur during this stage of acute exacerbation, and immediate

treatment is imperative. The pars tensa is reddened and inflamed. The surface epithelium of the tympanic membrane is thickened and whitish. There is a posterosuperior marginal perforation and a small epitympanic perforation. The stapes head appears on the medial wall of the pars tensa perforation, and there is necrotic epithelial debris within the perforation lumen.

Pars Flaccida, Acquired Cholesteatomas

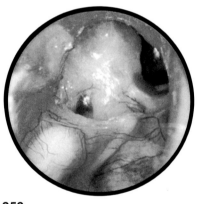

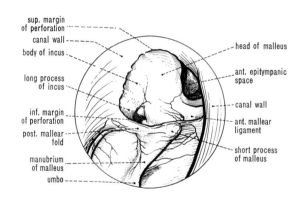

253

253a

253 Cholesteatoma, pars flaccida with natural atticotomy, right

The notch of Rivinus and the lateral epitympanic wall are eroded to expose the malleus head and a portion of the body of the incus. – This ear represents spontaneous

marsupialization of an epitympanic cholesteatoma which has resulted in a natural atticotomy. The cholesteatoma cyst has evacuated spontaneously, stopping further erosion and extension into the mastoid. – In Fig. **234** similar pathology is shown in a macrosection.

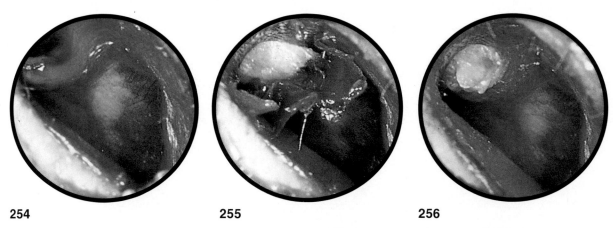

254   **255**   **256**

254 Cholesteatoma, pars flaccida, left
There is a small mass of what appears to be cerumen in the pars flaccida region.

255 Same ear as Figs 254 and 256
The cerumen has been carefully lifted away.

256 Same ear as Figs 254 and 255
The crust of cerumen and necrotic epithelial debris has been removed to expose a perforation of the pars flaccida filled with necrotic epithelial debris. A perforation such as this, filled with necrotic debris, is pathognomonic for a pars flaccida cholesteatoma.

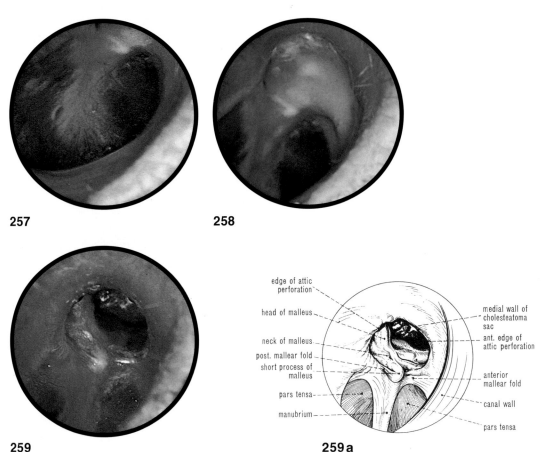

257   **258**

259   **259a**

257 Cholesteatoma, pars flaccida, right
The pars tensa is intact and the middle ear is air-filled. Just above the short process of the malleus there is a suspicious area.

258 Same ear as Figs 257 and 259
Training the otoscope superiorly shows a large epitympanic slough filled with purulent debris. The notch of Rivinus is eroded.

259 Same ear as Figs 257 and 258
The epithelial debris and purulent secretion are aspirated to expose a large, deep epitympanic perforation. The neck, part of the malleus head and cholesteatoma matrix are visible within the epitympanum. – These photographs demonstrate the importance of visualizing the entire tympanic membrane including the pars flaccida area, otherwise epitympanic lesions such as this would be overlooked.

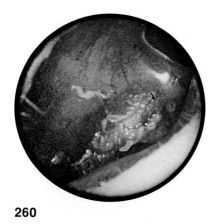

260

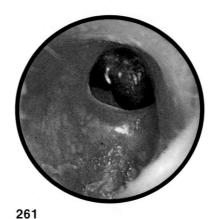

261

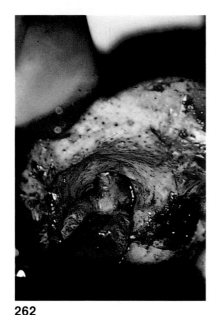

262

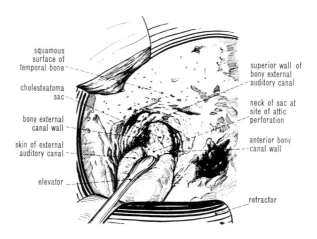

squamous
surface of
temporal bone

cholesteatoma
sac

bony external
canal wall

skin of external
auditory canal

elevator

superior wall of
bony external
auditory canal

neck of sac at
site of attic
perforation

anterior bony
canal wall

retractor

262a

260 Cholesteatoma, pars flaccida, right
The chronic purulent discharge that filled the external
auditory canal was removed prior to photography. The
pars tensa is somewhat inflamed. The malleus handle is
obscured by epithelial debris. A cursory examination
would overlook the small semilunar fold anterosuperiorly.

261 Same ear as Figs 260 and 262–264
When the otoscope is directed superiorly, a large
epitympanic perforation with erosion of the notch of
Rivinus is noted. The pus and epithelial debris which

filled the lumen of the perforation have been aspirated,
though some white epithelial debris is still visible in the
depths of the perforation.

**262 Same ear as Figs 260, 261, 263, and 264, surgical
pathology**
The skin of the external auditory canal has been dissected and depressed inferiorly to show the external appearance of the mouth of the cholesteatoma sac seen in Fig.
261. The epithelium of the cholesteatoma sac is continuous with the epithelium of the external auditory
canal.

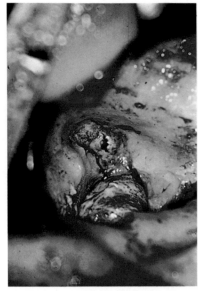

263

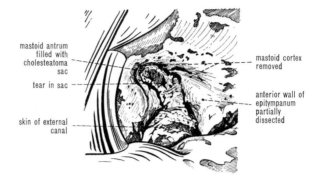

mastoid antrum
filled with
cholesteatoma
sac

tear in sac

skin of external
canal

mastoid cortex
removed

anterior wall of
epitympanum
partially
dissected

263 a

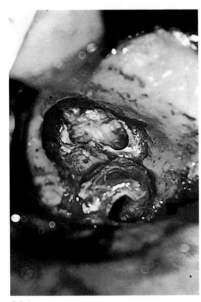

264

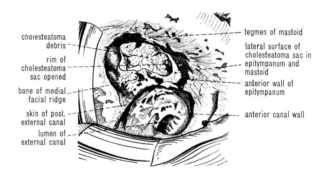

cholesteatoma
debris

rim of
cholesteatoma
sac opened

bone of medial
facial ridge

skin of post.
external canal

lumen of
external canal

tegmen of mastoid

lateral surface of
cholesteatoma sac in
epitympanum and
mastoid

anterior wall of
epitympanum

anterior canal wall

264 a

263 Same ear as Figs 260–262 and 264, surgical pathology

The superior wall of the bony external canal, the lateral epitympanic wall and the thickened overlying mastoid bone have been drilled away to show extension of the cholesteatoma sac into the mastoid antral area.

264 Same ear as Figs 260–263, surgical pathology

The sclerotic mastoid bone overlying the antrum has been drilled away, and the cholesteatoma partially opened to demonstrate the sac-like nature of the cholesteatoma. Necrotic epithelial debris fills the sac lumen. The malleus head and incus body have been eroded by the cholesteatoma.

Cholesteatomas with Aural Polyps

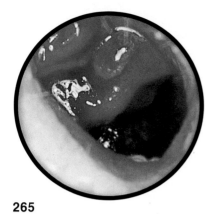

265

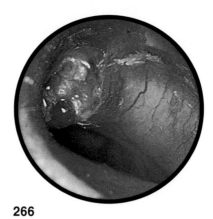

266

265 Cholesteatoma, pars flaccida with polyp, left
A large polyp fills the upper portion of the external auditory canal. The polyp was carefully removed and the ear treated with topical antibiotic and steroid medication. There was an erosion of the notch of Rivinus and epithelial debris in the lumen of the perforation. The polyp arose from granulation tissue in the epitympanum. Polyps of this type are characteristic of epitympanic cholesteatomas.

266 Cholesteatoma, pars flaccida with extension into middle ear, left
The epitympanic perforation is filled with necrotic epithelial debris, and there is a small granuloma at the inferior rim of the perforation. Extension of the cholesteatoma into the middle ear is seen lying on the medial surface of the intact posterosuperior quadrant of the pars tensa.

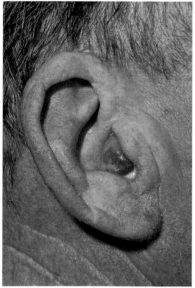

267

267 Cholesteatoma with aural polyp, right
This 65-year-old patient has had a foul-smelling otorrhea since childhood. Polyps had been removed twice in the past, but continued to form because the cholesteatoma of the mastoid was never treated. Since otoscopy is impossible when the polyp fills the entire canal, preoperative tomography is indicated to define the extent of the cholesteatoma. Biopsy showed chronic inflammation.

Primary Cholesteatoma, Cholesteatoma without Tympanic Membrane Perforation

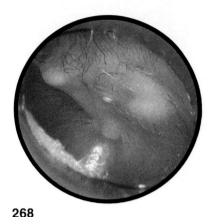

268

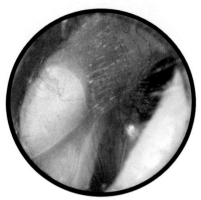

269

268 Cholesteatoma, primary, congenital with intact tympanic membrane, left

Behind the posterosuperior quadrant of the intact tympanic membrane of a four-year-old child, there is a whitish mass lying within the middle ear. The lesion was noted and diagnosed as probable cholesteatoma during microscopic otoscopy. – Despite being barely visible, at surgery there was a 0.7 cm cholesteatoma in the epitympanum which extended into the mastoid antrum. The long process of the incus was destroyed. – The pathogenesis of this cholesteatoma was most probably from an embryonic rest of stratified squamous epithelium in the epitympanum or antrum. – In the dif-

ferential diagnosis of this lesion, a herniated abnormal facial nerve, a meningomyelocele and connective tissue sarcoma were considered.

269 Cholesteatoma, congenital with intact tympanic membrane, right

In the posterior half of this middle ear, there is a whitish mass lying in contact with the medial surface of the tympanic membrane. The middle ear is air-filled anterior to the mass. There was no perforation of the tympanic membrane, and the assumption is that this cholesteatoma developed from an embryological rest. The patient is six years old.

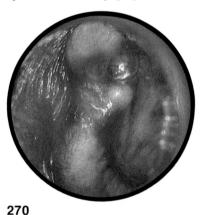

270

270 Cholesteatoma, pars flaccida area, without perforation, right

The notch of Rivinus is somewhat eroded. Above the short process of the malleus there is a dead white mass of necrotic desquamated epithelial debris lying underneath the intact pars flaccida. The otoscopic appearance leads one to suspect cholesteatoma. At surgery, the patient had a cholesteatoma extending into the epitympanum and eroding the horizontal semicircular canal. – The origin of this cholesteatoma cannot be determined. This lesion may be an example of a papillary cholesteatoma. Papillary downgrowth from the epidermis of the pars flaccida encysts to form a cholesteatoma. Once formed, the cyst enlarges and extends due to accumulated epithelial debris. – Otoscopically the extent of this lesion could not be determined, but tomography showed destruction of malleus and incus and fistulization of the horizontal semicircular canal.

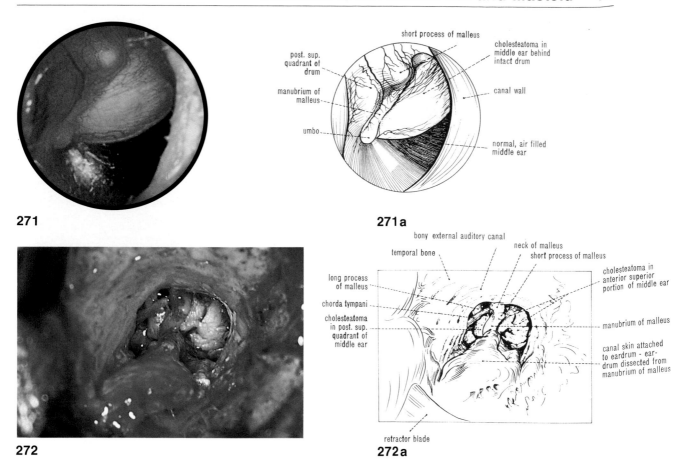

271

271a

272

272a

271 Cholesteatoma behind intact tympanic membrane, primary, congenital cholesteatoma, right
This four-year-old child had a whitish mass of cholesteatoma behind the intact anterosuperior quadrant of the tympanic membrane. The short process and handle of the malleus border the lesion posteriorly. The uninvolved portion of the middle ear is intact and there is no retraction or abnormality of the pars flaccida.

272 Same ear as Fig. 271, surgical pathology
The tympanic membrane has been dissected from the malleus handle and retracted inferiorly in continuity with the skin of the upper portion of the external auditory canal. The bony external canal has been enlarged. – The cholesteatomatous mass lies in the middle ear, medial to the malleus handle, and fills most of the anterior portion of the middle ear. – The incus long process and chorda tympani are normal and lie in the posterosuperior quadrant.

Traumatic and Iatrogenic Cholesteatomas

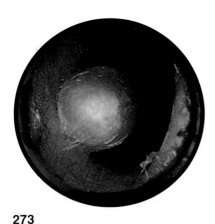

273 Cholesteatoma, external auditory canal, post-stapedectomy, right
Four months previously this patient underwent a stapedectomy for otosclerosis. This 4 mm epithelial cyst lies at the lateral extent of the endomeatal canal incision and was caused by inversion of a small bit of stratified squamous epithelium during surgery.

273

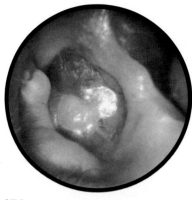

274

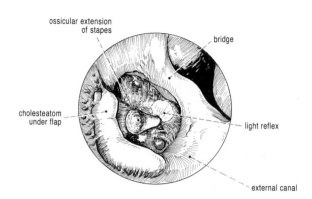

274a

ossicular extension of stapes

bridge

cholesteatom under flap

light reflex

external canal

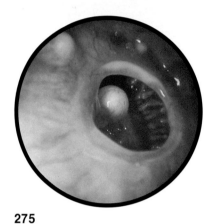

275

274 Cholesteatoma, iatrogenic, in tympanomeatal graft, left

Following tympanoplasty, the ossicular extension of the stapes lies in contact with the tympanic membrane graft. The graft has retracted into the antrum above the intact mastoid bridge. There is a large cholesteatoma cyst on the anteroinferior canal wall under the overlay graft that was applied to this area.

275 Traumatic cholesteatoma, right

This Iraqi soldier was wounded by a mine which blew off his right leg and perforated his right tympanic membrane. A small cholesteatoma has formed on the promontory due to medial displacement of stratified squamous epithelium by the blast injury. The malleus short process lies at 11 o'clock and the cyst lies just anterior to the umbo. (Patient supine.)

Otosclerosis

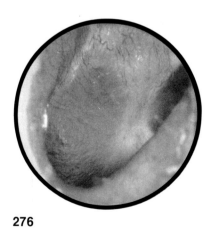

276

Otosclerosis, Schwartze's sign, right

The patient has otosclerosis with a mixed deafness. There is a red blush of the promontory seen through the translucent posterior portion of the tympanic membrane. This blush is due to hyperemia of the mucosa overlying the vascular otosclerotic focus on the promontory. – See Figs **277** and **278** for the tomographic appearance of a similar ear with Schwartze's sign. The tomography demonstrates severe demineralization of the cochlea. – Schwartze's sign is a rare finding and usually indicates presence of red, vascular malignant otosclerosis. This type of otosclerosis is characterized by rapid progression and severe sensorineural deafness.

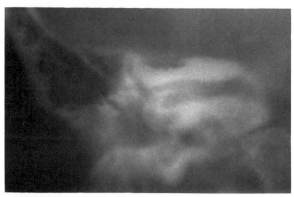

277

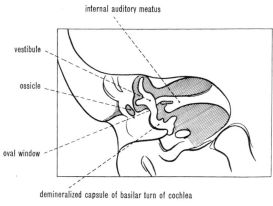

internal auditory meatus

vestibule

ossicle

oval window

demineralized capsule of basilar turn of cochlea

277 a

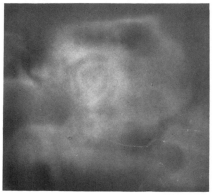

278

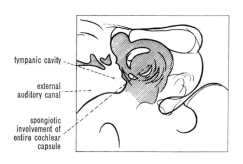

tympanic cavity

external
auditory canal

spongiotic
involvement of
entire cochlear
capsule

278 a

277 Cochlear otosclerosis
Frontal tomogram of the right ear, showing severe demineralization of the capsule of the basilar turn of the
cochlea, which has lost its normal sharpness.

278 Cochlear otosclerosis
Frontal tomogram of the right ear, showing diffuse
spongiotic involvement of the entire cochlear capsule.
See normal tomographic findings at these levels in Figs
98–100.

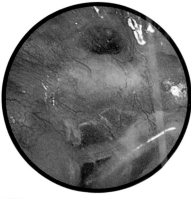

279

**279 Otoscopic findings of the Lempert fenestra nov-
ovalis, right**
This is the otoscopic appearance of an ear in which the
Lempert fenestra novovalis has been performed. The
camera is directed posterosuperiorly and focuses on the
fenestra in the horizontal semicircular canal. The fenestra is the darkened oval area in the upper part of the
photograph and lies above the facial nerve. Below the
facial nerve the tympanomeatal flap stretches laterally
over the chorda tympani onto the tympanic membrane.
The malleus short process and handle are visible at the
lower right.

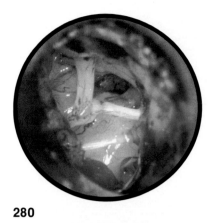

280

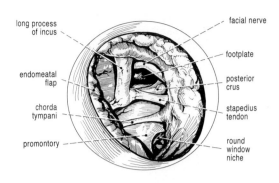

280a

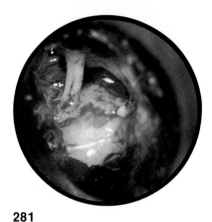

281

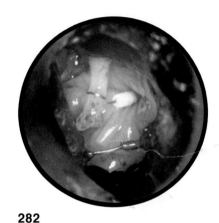

282

280 Otosclerosis, stapedectomy with Schuknecht stapes prosthesis, left

The endomeatal flap is retracted anteriorly. The round window lies inferior to the stapes and stapedius tendon. The posterior crus of the stapes and the thin footplate are seen inferior to the facial nerve. The long process of the incus is attached to the stapes.

281 Same ear as Figs 280 and 282

The stapes has been removed, and there is a light reflex from the perilymph in the vestibule. There is a minute amount of blood at the anterior margin of the footplate.

282 Same ear as Figs 280 and 281

The tef-wire prosthesis is now in place and crimped to the long process of the incus. The oval window has been covered with a 4 x 6 mm vein graft.

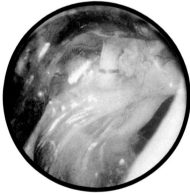

283

283 Otosclerosis, post-stapedectomy, right

The wire loop of a stapes prosthesis is attached to the long process of the incus. The posterosuperior quadrant of the tympanic membrane is somewhat atrophic and retracted and allows visualization of the metal loop.

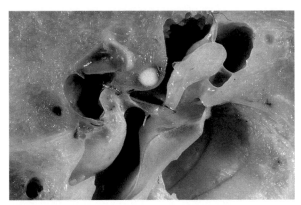

284

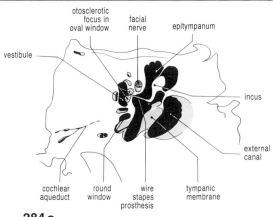

284 a

284 Otosclerosis, post-stapedectomy, coronal cross section

This coronal cross section crosses the oval window, middle ear, and epitympanum. The view looks from the posterior toward the anterior portion of the middle ear

and shows a wire stapes prosthesis extending into the oval window and attached to the long process of the incus. The utricle lies in the upper portion of the vestibule, and the round window opens into the round window niche.

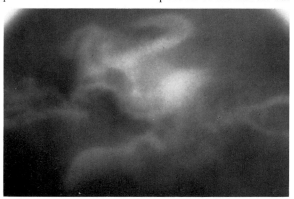

285

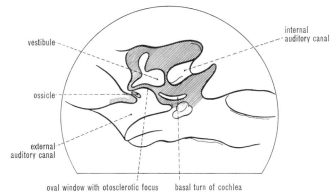

285 a

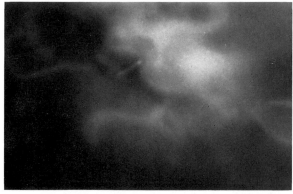

286

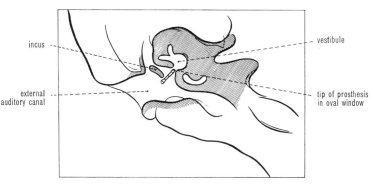

286 a

285 Fenestral otosclerosis

Frontal tomogram of the right ear, showing complete obliteration of the oval window by a thick footplate of the stapes.

286 Same ear as Fig. 286 after stapedectomy

Frontal tomogram of the same ear after stapedectomy, showing a fully reopened oval window and a metallic prosthesis extending from it to the long process of the incus. The fat and wire technique was used.

Glomus Tumors (Nonchromaffin Paragangliomas, Chemodectomas) and Differential Diagnosis

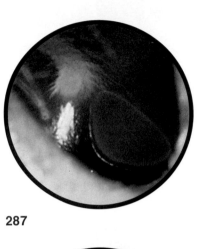

287

287 Glomus tumor, left

A small glomus tumor lies in the posteroinferior quadrant of the middle ear in contact with a normal, intact tympanic membrane. A fine refractile white line outlines the contact of the tumor on the medial surface of the membrane. – In addition to this lesion, the patient had a separate lesion in the jugular foramen which caused paralysis of the ninth, tenth, eleventh, and twelfth cranial nerves.

288 Glomus tumor, same ear as Fig. 287, surgical findings

Elevation of an endomeatal flap exposes the glomus tumor on the promontory. The tumor lies in relation to the tympanic nerve. – Radiographic studies of the temporal bone are essential in the evaluation of glomus tumors. Tomography is indispensable and often venography and arteriography are indicated.

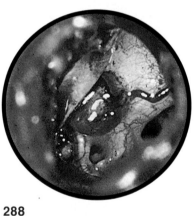

288

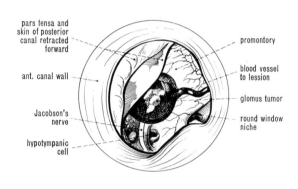

288 a

pars tensa and skin of posterior canal retracted forward

promontory

ant. canal wall

blood vessel to lession

glomus tumor

Jacobson's nerve

round window niche

hypotympanic cell

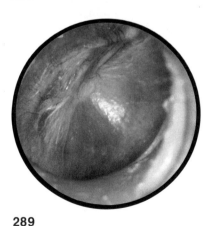

289

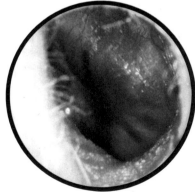

290

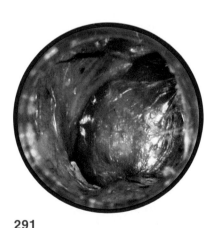

291

289 Glomus tumor, right

This glomus tumor, extending from the floor of the middle ear, reaches the level of the umbo behind a normal tympanic membrane.

290 Glomus tumor, left

A glomus tumor fills the posterior half of the middle ear and causes a lateral bulge of the intact tympanic membrane.

291 Glomus tumor, right

A large glomus tumor has extended through the tympanic membrane into the external auditory canal. The lesion has the characteristic deep red-blue color of a glomus tumor which differentiates this lesion from a granulomatous ear polyp. This lesion pulsed synchronously with the heartbeat. – When biopsying an aural polyp suspected of being a glomus tumor, the surgeon must be prepared to control hemorrhage.

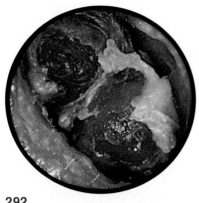

292

292 Glomus tumor, left
A large bilobed glomus tumor arising from the jugular fossa fills the lumen of the external auditory canal. The tumor has sloughed the tympanic membrane.

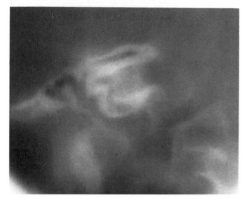

293

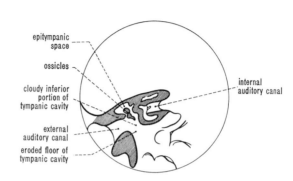

293 a

293 Glomus jugulare tumor
Semiaxial tomogram of the right ear, showing clouding of the lower half of the tympanic cavity by a soft tissue mass and destruction of the inferior wall of the hypotympanum.

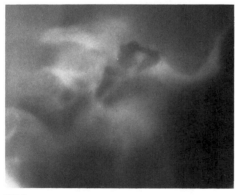

294

294 a

294 Normal ear
Corresponding semiaxial view of the normal left ear for comparison.

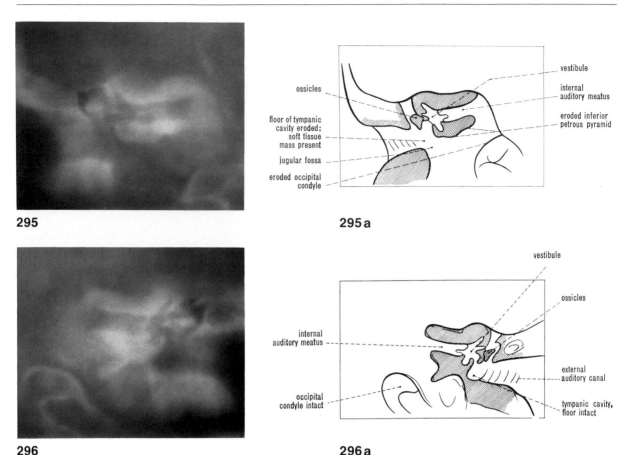

295

295a

296

296a

295 Glomus jugulare tumor
Frontal tomogram of the right ear, showing enlargement of the jugular fossa with destruction of the inferior aspect of the petrous pyramid including the inferior wall of the tympanic cavity and erosion of the adjacent portion of the occipital condyle.

296 Normal ear
Corresponding frontal tomogram of normal left ear.

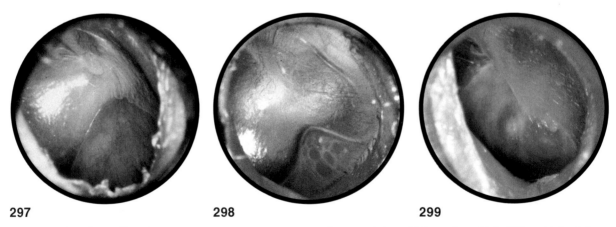

297   **298**   **299**

297 High jugular bulb, left
The dome of the jugular bulb projects high into the posteroinferior portion of the middle ear. The jugular vein has no bony cover and lies in contact with the medial surface of the normal tympanic membrane. – The deep blue color of the jugular vein in this minor anomaly differentiates it from glomus tumor and an ectopic internal carotid artery.

298 Glomus tumor, left
A small glomus tumor projects into the posterior inferior portion of the middle ear. The tumor has the characteristic red-blue color which differentiates it from a high jugular bulb, Fig. **297**, and an ectopic internal carotid, Fig. **299**.

299 Ectopic internal carotid artery, left
A deep red purple mass lies in contact with the medial surface of the inferior portion of the normal tympanic membrane. Tomography and arteriography differentiate this lesion from a glomus tumor, Fig. **298**, and high jugular bulb, Fig. **297**. – Attempted biopsy of an ectopic internal carotid artery can lead to massive hemorrhage and severe neurological complications.

Diseases of the Face, Salivary Glands, External Nose

Diseases of the Face

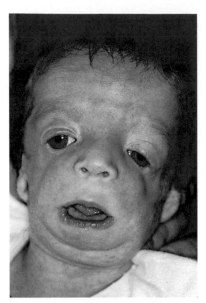

300

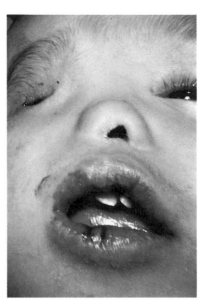

301

300 Franceschetti syndrome, mandibulofacial dysostosis

The syndrome is characterized by an antimongoloid lid axis, a lower lid coloboma, hypoplasia of the maxilla and zygoma, microgenia, a large fishlike mouth, and auricle and external auditory canal dysplasias. Varying degrees of these deformities occur in individual cases.

301 Nasal dysplasia, Klein-Waardenburg syndrome

The syndrome is an autosomal recessive complex causing congenital anomalies. There is nasal dystrophy, unilateral defect of the eye, hypertelorism, a white forelock, and congenital deafness. The mother and grandfather of the child had a rudiment of the syndrome in the form of a white forelock and congenital deafness.

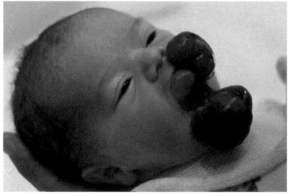

302

302 Congenital myoblastic myoma

This newborn female has huge, multiple firm brown red tumors arising from the upper and lower dental lamina. The lesions were removed surgically. Histologic examination showed a benign myoblastic myoma.

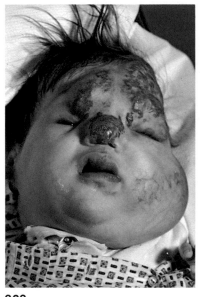

303

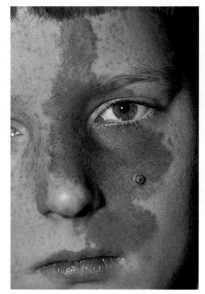

304

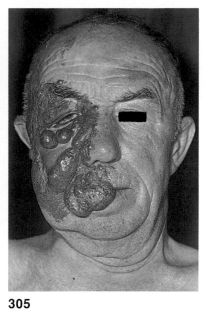

305

303–305 Craniofacial vascular nevus
This congenital syndrome (Sturge-Weber) is characterized by glaucomatous eye involvement associated with a nevus whose distribution corresponds to that of the trigeminal nerve. The brain lesions are occipital and parietal pial angiomas, which tend to calcify. The distribution of multiple angiomas about the head of the

12-week-old infant shown in Fig. **303** is typical of many combinations of encephalofacial angiomatosis. Fig. **304** shows an incidental pyogenic granuloma on the left cheek bone near the margin of a large facial hemangioma. Fig. **305** shows a unilateral cavernous hemangioma on the right side of the face.

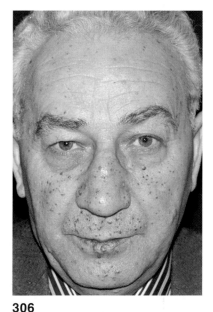

306

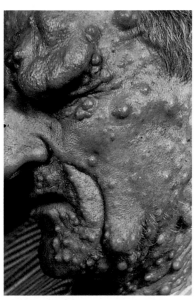

307

306 Weber-Rendu-Osler's disease
There are multiple, well-defined telangiectasias in the upper and lower lips, the cheeks, and the nose. The patient has similar lesions on the tongue, the nasopharynx, and larynx. Frequent epistaxis leads to severe anemia.

307 Generalized neurofibromatosis, Recklinghausen's disease
This patient has an unusually severe number of neurofibromas of the face. There is elephantiasis of the upper eyelid.

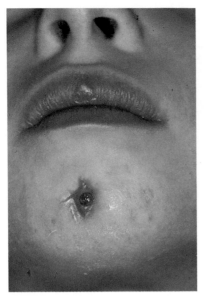

308

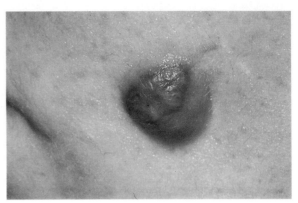

309

308 Dentigerous fistula of the chin
In this case, as in Fig. **309,** actinomycosis should be considered in the differential diagnosis. Actinomycosis, however, causes multiple fistuli and woody, hard swelling in the surrounding area.

309 Dentigerous fistula of the cheek
An earlier operation for a parotid fistula was unsuccessful because the origin of the fistula was a granuloma of the first upper left molar. Following excision of the entire fistulous tract and extraction of the affected tooth, the lesion healed. The corner of the left side of the mouth appears at the left in the photo.

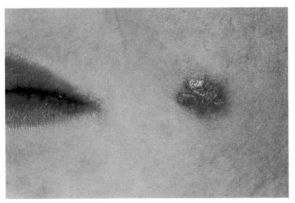

310

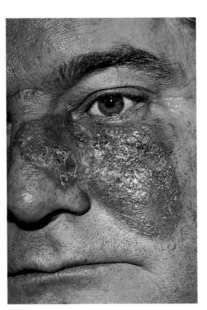

311

310 Lupus vulgaris
Under pressure by a glass spatula or slide this lesion shows the characteristic brownish, apple-jelly color of cutaneous tuberculosis of this lesion of the cheek. These lesions are characteristically soft to palpation.

311 Lupus vulgaris of the face
There is a characteristic red-brown infiltration and edema with central scaling in this tuberculosis of the skin of the face. Pressure on the lesion with a glass slide reveals the apple-jelly color of the tubercular lesion. When probed, the lesions are soft and fragile.

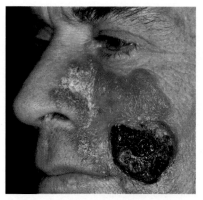

312

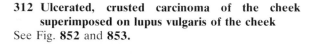

312 Ulcerated, crusted carcinoma of the cheek superimposed on lupus vulgaris of the cheek
See Fig. **852** and **853**.

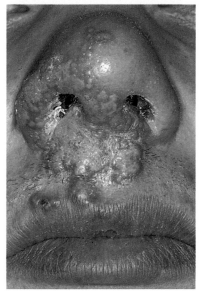

313

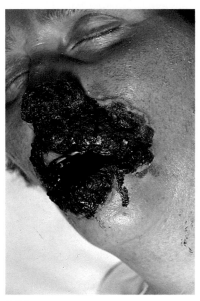

314

313 Herpes simplex
The herpes lesions involve the upper lip and nostril to an unusually widespread degree.

314 Herpes simplex
A rare variant of herpes simplex in the presence of anergy occurs as the aphthoid of Pospischill-Feyrter. This patient had an aplastic anemia. The clotted blood which covers the surface of the lesion is due to a bleeding tendency. The characteristic gyrate vesicular margin appears on the cheek.

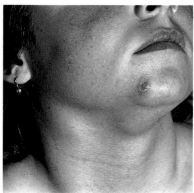

315

315 Cat scratch fever
This is the typical appearance of a late primary lesion on the chin with regional submental and submandibular lymphadenitis. The diagnostic Mollaret-Debré skin test was strongly positive.

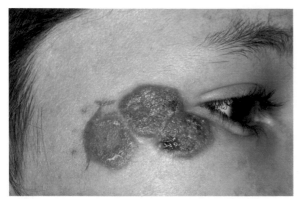

316

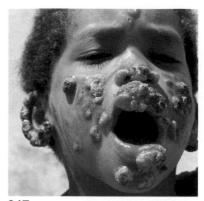

317

316 Cutaneous leishmaniasis, oriental boil
This thirteen-year-old Syrian patient has cutaneous leishmaniasis of the old world type, known as the oriental boil. Parasites were found in the biopsy. Lesions such as this usually heal slowly over a period of one year with scarring.

317 Cutaneous leishmaniasis
A lepromatous form of Leishmania braziliensis (new world type) is present in this ten-year-old boy. The granulomas are laden with leishmania parasites. This disorder typically is resistant to therapy.

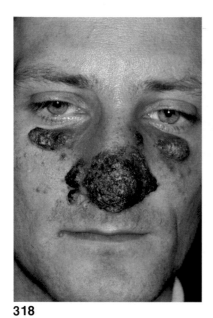

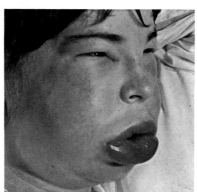

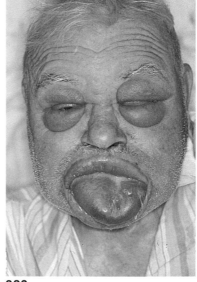

318   **319**   **320**

318 Iododerma vegetans
These lesions followed long term use of an iodine containing syrup for bronchial asthma.

319 Angioneurotic facial edema
Particularly apparent is the orbital and labial edema in addition to the diffuse facial swelling affecting the areolar tissues. In some instances, typified in this patient, there is a familial history of recurring edema (Quincke) which may also affect the intraoral and hypopharyngeal areas, in which case airway obstruction may pose a problem. – Edematous contact dermatitis can be ruled out by the rather smooth appearance of these angioneurotic lesions (see fig. **659**).

320 Edema of the face secondary to venous and lymphatic obstruction
There was an extensive carcinoma of the base of the tongue with extension into the epiglottis in this 68-year-old patient. He was treated with laryngectomy, resection of the base of the tongue, and bilateral radical neck dissection.

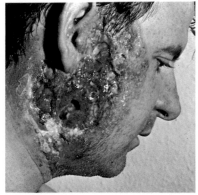

321

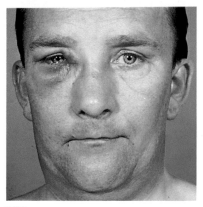

321 Pyoderma gangrenosum of the face
This lesion occurred in conjunction with ulcerative colitis.

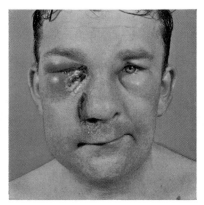

322

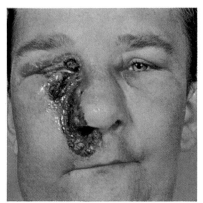

323   **324**

322–324 Midline lethal granuloma
In this 39-year-old patient there was a two-year history of nasal obstruction, purulent nasal discharge, and occasional epistaxis. Redding of the skin below the eye and at the side of the nose over a period of one month developed into a painless ulceration, and this progressed to destruction of the columella, the anterior nasal septum, the lateral nasal wall, and the palate. – The gangrenous lethal midline granuloma is a destructive lesion involving the nostrils, the paranasal sinuses, the palate, and the pharynx. – A differential diagnosis of this lesion must be made from Wegener's granuloma, malignant lymphoma, leukemia or agranulocytic states. The photos here demonstrate the rapidly fatal course over a period of four months.

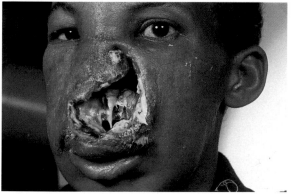

325

325 Noma
There is a rapidly progressing fatal gangrene of the soft parts of the midface in this 25-year-old patient from Somalia.

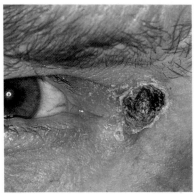

326

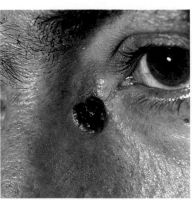

327

326 Basal cell carcinoma of the inner canthus, right eye
Basal cell carcinomas are locally malignant and over a period of time are locally destructive. They do not ordinarily metastasize.

327 Pigmented basal cell carcinoma of the inner canthus
This pigmented basal cell tumor, which contains a large amount of melanin, must be distinguished histologically from a malignant melanoma. The latter is less firm and bleeds readily on contact, see Fig. **57.**

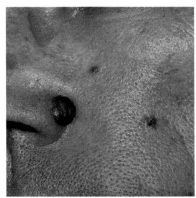

328

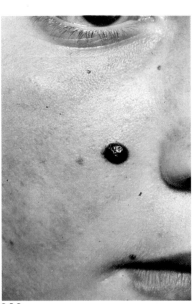

329

328 Pigmented basal cell carcinoma of the left ala nasi and cheek
This lesion occurred in a 49-year-old male. The clinical differential diagnosis of a pigmented basal cell carcinoma from a melanoma is difficult at times. Melanomas tend to be less firm and more destructive and mottled than the basal cell carcinoma. When a brown mole changes appearance and enlarges, the lesion is usually a melanoma. – Basal cell carcinomas usually are silent lesions while the melanomas are often pruritic, cause a burning sensation, and bleed easily. – The differential diagnosis in this case is especially difficult since the two additional pigmented basal cell lesions lateral to the carcinoma of the ala nasi appear to be almost pathognomonic for a malignant melanoma with cutaneous metastases, see Fig. **59.** However, in this case, biopsy showed small pigmented basal cell lesions.

329 Nevus cell nevus of the cheek
This benign lesion occurred in a young girl.

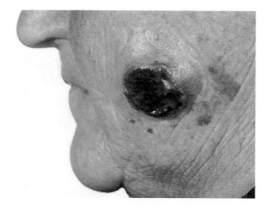

330

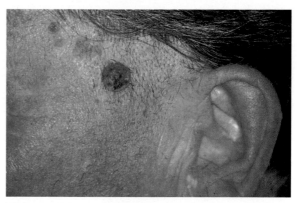

331

330 Nodular malignant melanoma
In this 79-year-old patient there was a rapid, six-month growth of this lesion of the left cheek. There were spontaneous bleeding, itching, and submandibular lymph node metastases.

331 Squamous cell carcinoma of the temporal region
This 73-year-old patient noted a gradually enlarging "wart" on his left temple. – There is a metastatic node at the hair line.

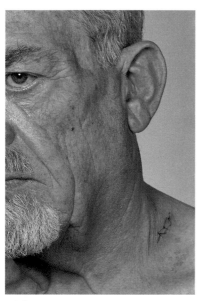

332

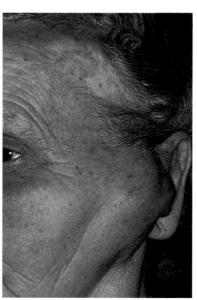

333

332–333 Squamous cell carcinoma with regional lymph node metastases
In the 67-ear-old patient in Fig. **332** a squamous cell carcinoma from the skin of the temple was removed and the patient irradiated with 5000 rads six months previously. The radiodermatitis of the skin is visible. The patient stated that a few weeks prior to photography he felt nodes below the site of the original lesion. Examination showed metastases in the parotid, upper jugular, cervi-

cal, and supraclavicular areas. Biopsy showed squamous metastatic carcinoma. Note the sutures at the biopsy site. – Fig. **333** shows a 75-year-old female at first suspected to have an ulcerating parotid carcinoma. When the hair of the temple was retracted radiodermatitis was discovered. A more careful history revealed that a squamous cell carcinoma of the temple was treated locally with radiotherapy some years before which led to the ulcerative metastases in the parotid.

Diseases of the Salivary Glands

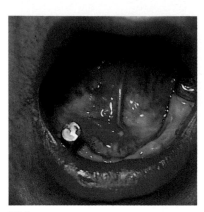

334

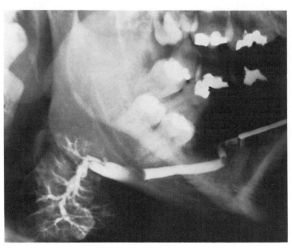

335

334–335 Sialolith, Wharton's duct, right
This patient noted pain below the tongue and in the right submandibular region while eating. In the sublingual caruncle there is a small drop of pus. The inflammation and swelling of the submandibular duct indicate the presence of a sialolith in Wharton's duct. The subman-

dibular gland was firm and tender, Fig. **334.** When salivary stones contain calcium they can be visualized directly on a radiograph. – At times sialography is needed to visualize the stones, as in Fig. **335.** There is a large radiolucent stone in the mid-portion of the duct and a smaller stone at the caruncle just distal to the cannula.

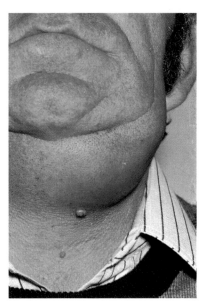

336

336 Submandibular abscess, left
For one month the patient noted pain and swelling of the submandibular gland while eating. An abscess has formed, secondary to sialolithiasis.

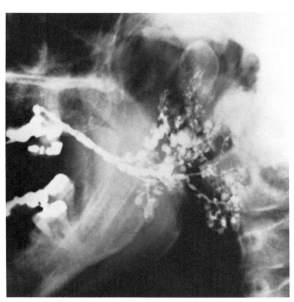

337

337 Chronic recurrent parotitis
The sialogram demonstrates the typical changes of chronic parotitis. Beading of the main ducts and dilatation of the acini area especially noteworthy.

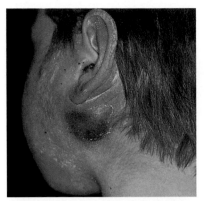

338

338 Postoperative suppurative parotitis
Abdominal surgery for a ruptured appendix was compli-cated by peritonitis in this patient. Secondary phleg-monous parotitis occurred followed by abscess forma-tion and a breakthrough into the external auditory canal by way of the fissure of Santorini.

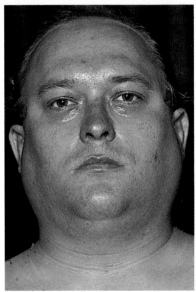

339

339 Sialadenosis of the parotid
Differentiation is necessary between an inflammatory state and neoplastic swelling of the gland as contrasted with bilateral, painless enlargement. In the latter condi-tion, involvement of the salivary gland, especially the parotid, reflects a generalized disease entity such as en-docrine, metabolic or neurogenic disorders or drug reac-tions. The patient shown here is a 30-year-old wine grower who had bilateral non-inflammatory parotid swelling with subicteric hepatic cirrhosis.

Tumors

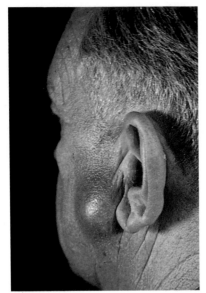

340

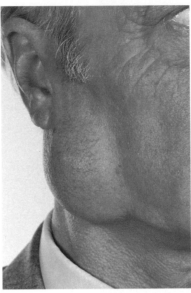

341

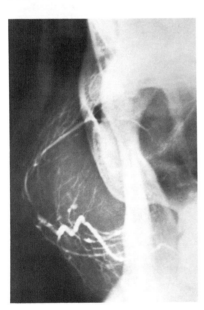

342

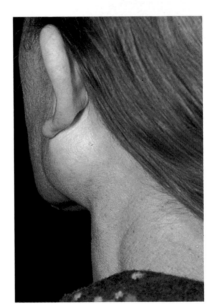

343

340–343 Pleomorphic adenoma, mixed tumor of the parotid

The site of predilection for mixed tumors is the parotid gland, usually in the lateral facial or superficial portion and rarely in the deep portion. Tumor growth occurs over a period of several years, even decades. The lesions are usually encapsulated and mobile, and they have a firm to hard consistency, and are nontender. These benign lesions do not cause facial paralysis since they stretch the nerve and do not infiltrate it. – Fig. **340** shows a 58-year-old male with a twelve-year history of a slowly growing, nontender mass, arising from the superficial portion of the parotid gland. – Fig. **341** is a 59-year-old with a similar ten-year history. – Sialography, Fig. **342,** shows the mass of the tumor outlined by the stretched parotid ducts. – Fig. **343** shows a 53-year-old female with a ten-year history of tumor growth. This lesion lies wedged between the mandibular ramus and the mastoid process, and caused difficulty in chewing. In the German literature it is known as an "iceberg tumor."

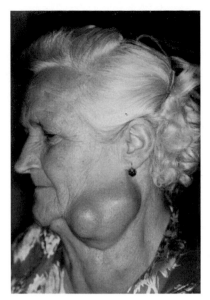

344

344 Lobulated pleomorphic adenoma, mixed tumor of the submaxillary gland
There was a history of slow tumor growth of more than twenty years.

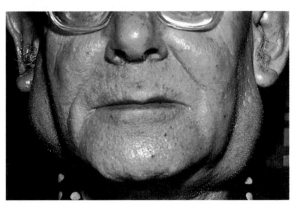

345

345 Papillary cystadenoma,
Warthin tumor of both parotid glands
These benign tumors grew slowly over a period of eight years in both parotid glands of this 59-year-old patient. – These lesions are often bilateral and occur more commonly in the inferior portion of the parotid gland.

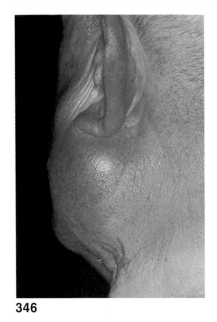

346

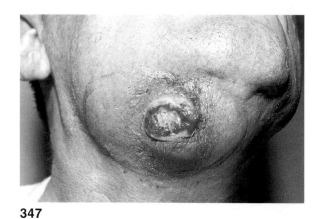

347

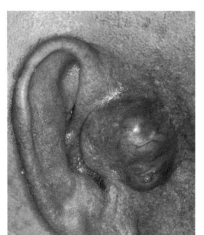

348

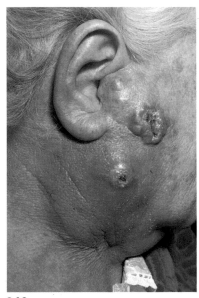

349

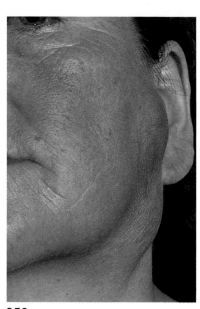

350

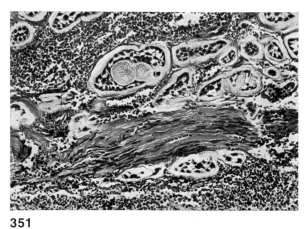

351

346–351 Salivary gland malignant tumors
Signs of malignancy in salivary gland tumors are:
Pain and infiltration of the skin, Fig. **346, 348;**
Ulceration of the overlying skin, Fig. **347, 349;**
Osteolysis of the adjacent bony structures, and regional lymph node metastases, Fig. **350.**
At times partial or complete paralysis of the facial nerve. Fig. **351,** histopathology of an adenocystic carcinoma showing extension of the tumor along the nerve fibers. In addition these lesions spread slowly into the connective tissue surrounding the affected gland and metastasize to lymph nodes and via the blood stream. Histologic and clinically malignant lesions include: carcinomas in pleomorphic adenomas, squamous and adenocarcinomas, mucoepidermoid carcinomas and acinar cell carcinomas.

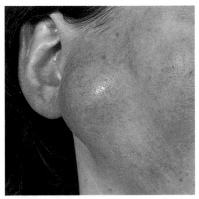

352

352 Lymphoblastic, non-Hodgkin lymphoma, right parotid gland

This 20-year-old female noted rapid growth of this lesion of her parotid gland accompanied by facial paralysis. Involvement of the parotid by non-Hodgkin lymphoma and other lymphoreticular system tumors is due to the extensive peri- and intraglandular lymph nodes.

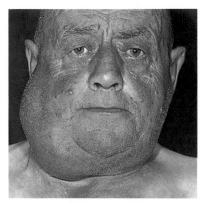

353

353 Lymphocytic, non-Hodgkin lymphoma, parotid and submaxillary lymph nodes

This 73-year-old patient noted a swelling in the region of the right parotid and submandibular glands over a period of eight weeks. Enlarged lymph nodes were found in the axilla and inguinal regions and were also demonstrated in the mediastinum.

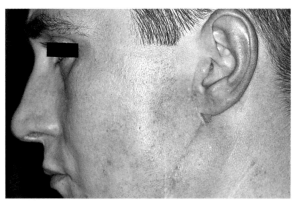

354

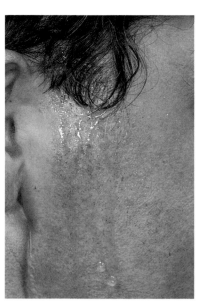

356

354–356 Auriculotemporal syndrome, Frey's syndrome, sweating and flushing syndrome

This syndrome can arise following parotid gland injury, infection, and most commonly surgical excision. There is a latent period of a few months to a few years before the syndrome manifests itself. In Figs **354** and **355** the patient had a parotidectomy for chronic parotitis with preservation of facial nerve function nine months previously. Before eating the parotid area is normal, Fig. **354,** but after eating, hyperhydrosis, erythema, and hyperesthesia occur in the overlying skin, Fig. **355**. The cause of this phenomenon may be a lesion of the auriculotemporal nerve. – Formes frustes of this syndrome are more common than the fullblown picture. In Fig. **356** sweat runs down the cheek from the temple area.

355

Diseases of the External Nose

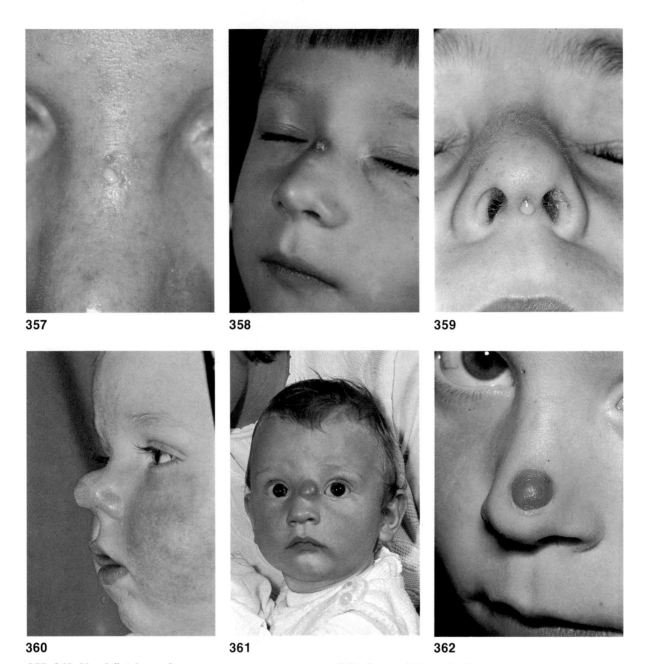

357

358

359

360

361

362

357–360 Nasal fistulas and cysts

Small, noninflamed or inflamed and suppurative congenital fistulas occur usually in the midline of the nose at various levels. Fig. **357** shows a quiescent lesion, and in Fig. **358** there is purulent discharge and perifistular skin inflammation. The fistula opens into the columella in Fig. **359**. – Midline nasal fistulas often extend to, and arise from, the dura of the anterior cranial fossa. – Fig. **360** shows a cyst in the nasal tip of a two-year-old child. At surgery a cyst filled with thick mucoid secretion and hair was found. The fistula tract extended between the nasal bones and reached the anterior cranial dura.

361 Congenital nasal glioma

The diagnosis is established histologically by the astrocytes seen in the glial fibers. There was no radiographic evidence of bone destruction, and at surgery the lesion was not attached to dura. The lesion can be classified as a choristoma.

362 Juvenile melanoma

This is a benign lesion histologically despite the term melanoma.

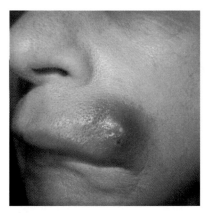

363

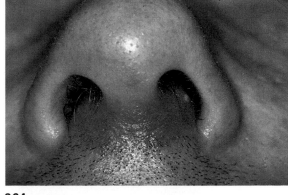

364

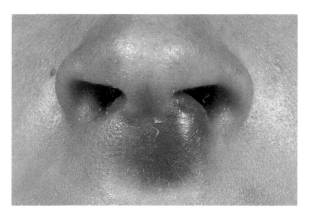

365

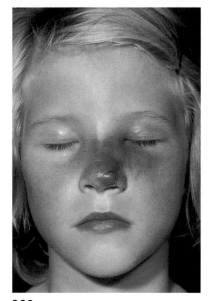

366

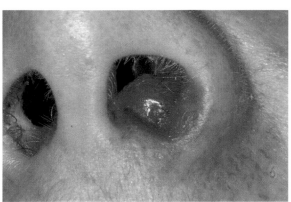

367

363–367 Furuncles of the upper lip and the nose
Different aspects of furuncles of the upper lip and the nose are shown here, Figs **363–365.** The frightful complication of these lesions, angular vein thrombosis, Fig. **366** and cavernous sinus thrombosis, are today extremely rare thanks to antibiotic treatment. – Fig. **367** shows a differential diagnostic problem. The patient had an **infected cyst of the nasal floor** that was treated as a furuncle for four weeks with antibiotics. The lesion failed to heal, the correct diagnosis was made and the lesion excised.

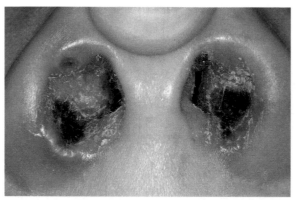

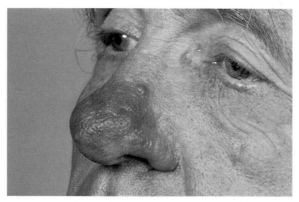

368

368 Vaccinia translata of the nostrils
This child inoculated her nose by carrying virus from the vaccination site on her arm to her nose with her fingers.

369

369 Early rhinophyma
The lesion arises from a chronic rosacea.

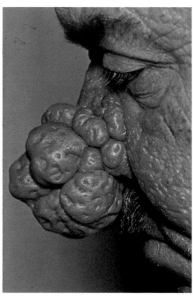

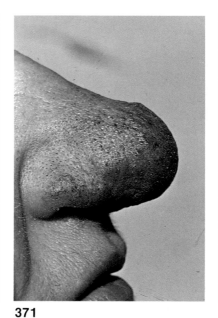

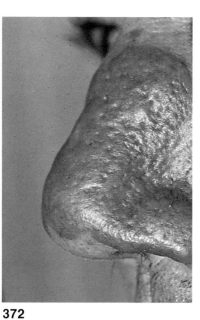

370   **371**   **372**

370 Rhinophyma
Rhinophyma, pound nose, occurs almost always in men, and arises from a preexisting rosacea.

371 Sarcoidosis of Besnier-Boeck-Schaumann
This is the typical appearance of lupus pernio with a nodular, cyanotic swelling of the nose. See Figs. **456 + 850.**

372 Eosinophilic facial granuloma
The nodular or plaquelike lesions, reddish to brownish yellow in color, are characterized by follicular dilatations and are found only in isolated foci of the facial region. There is no systemic involvement. Histologically, there is a polymorphic granuloma consisting of reticulum cells, plasma cells, eosinophilic leukocytes, and histiocytes with few giant cells.

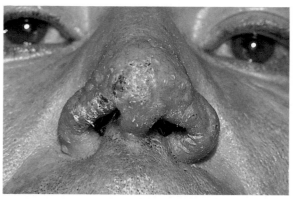

373

373 Lepromatous leprosy
In the lepromatous form of this disease, foci of nodular lepromatous lesions occur chiefly in the nasal region. Typical is the destruction of the nasal cartilage so that the nose appears flattened and widened (s. also Figs **38, 444, 846**).

Tumors

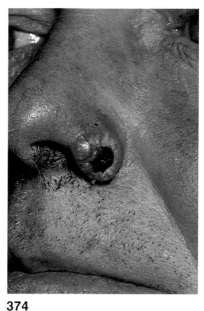

374

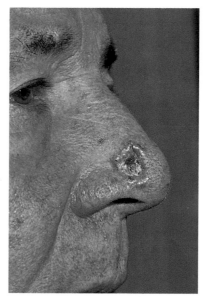

375

374 Keratoacanthoma of the nasal ala
The photo shows the typical appearance of an acanthoma.

375 Basal cell carcinoma, rodent ulcer
The gray red rolled margin of the lesion is typical.

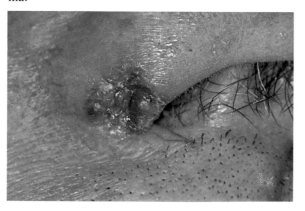

376

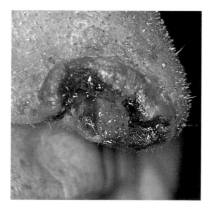

377

376 Basal cell carcinoma, rodent ulcer, nasal ala

377 Basal cell carcinoma, penetrating type, nasal ala
Despite the clinical appearance resembling a squamous cell carcinoma, biopsy showed a basal cell lesion.

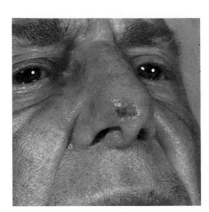

378

378 Squamous cell carcinoma of the nasal tip

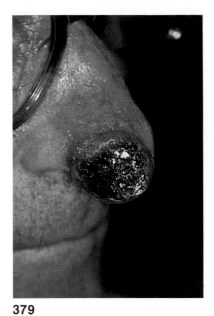

379

379 Squamous cell carcinoma of the nasal ala
Despite a three-month history, this lesion is associated with metastases to the submandibular and submental lymph nodes.

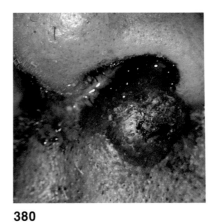

380

380 Squamous cell carcinoma of the nasal vestibule
There is beginning ulceration.

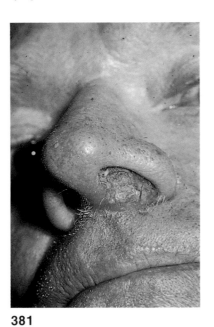

381

381 Squamous cell carcinoma of the nasal vestibule

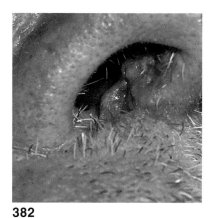

382

382 **Squamous cell carcinoma of the right nasal columella**

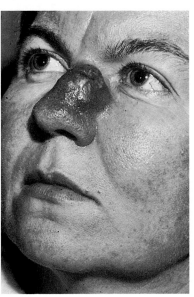

383

383 **Squamous cell carcinoma of the nose**
There are submandibular metastases. The yellowish ointment on the surface of the lesion was used by the patient for many weeks in a vain attempt to treat the "sore".

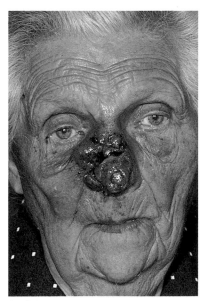

384

384 **Squamous cell carcinoma of the nose**
For three years this 90-year-old female patient had noted a "sore", which started on the right side of the nose. The carcinoma destroyed the bony and cartilaginous dorsum of the nose as well as large portions of the septum and invaded the perinasal skin.

Diseases of the Inner Nose and Paranasal Sinuses

Roentgen and Clinical Anatomy of the Nose and Paranasal Sinuses

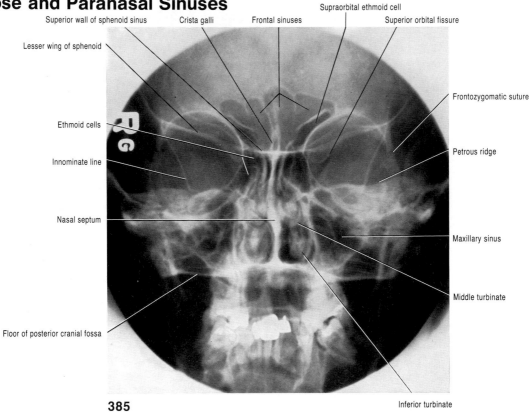

Superior wall of sphenoid sinus — Crista galli — Frontal sinuses — Supraorbital ethmoid cell — Superior orbital fissure

Lesser wing of sphenoid

Ethmoid cells

Innominate line

Nasal septum

Floor of posterior cranial fossa

Frontozygomatic suture

Petrous ridge

Maxillary sinus

Middle turbinate

Inferior turbinate

385

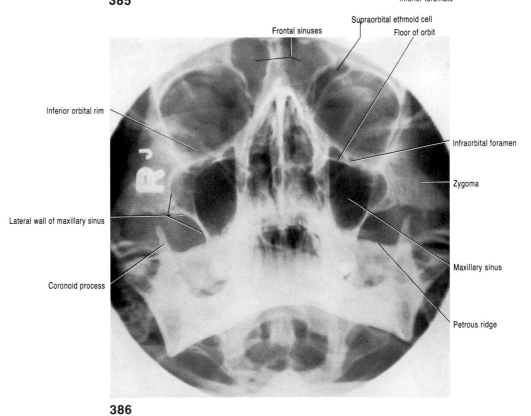

Frontal sinuses — Supraorbital ethmoid cell — Floor of orbit

Inferior orbital rim

Lateral wall of maxillary sinus

Coronoid process

Infraorbital foramen

Zygoma

Maxillary sinus

Petrous ridge

386

385 Caldwell projection
Patient faces the film, his nose and forehead touching the cassette holder.

386 Waters projection
Patient faces the film, his chin touching the cassette holder.

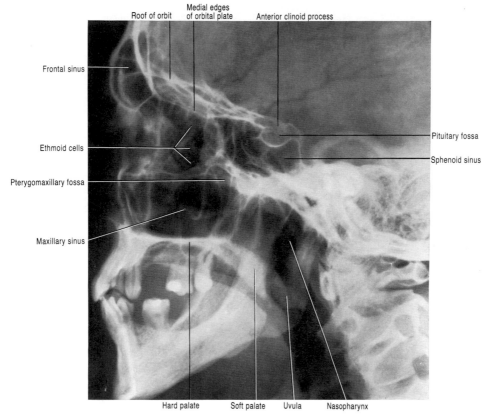

387

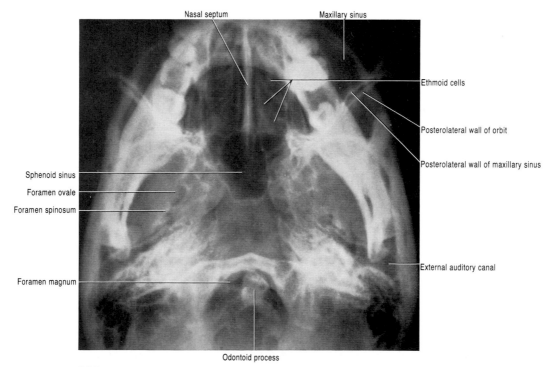

388

387 Lateral projection
The medial sagittal plane of the skull is parallel to the film. The central x-ray beam is directed perpendicular to the film to a point midway between the outer canthus and the external auditory canal.

388 Basal or axial projection
The neck is hyperextended so that the orbital meatal plane is parallel to the film. The medial sagittal plane of the skull and the central x-ray beam are perpendicular to the film.

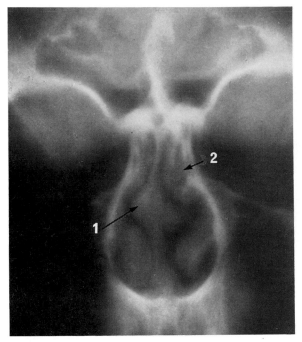

389a

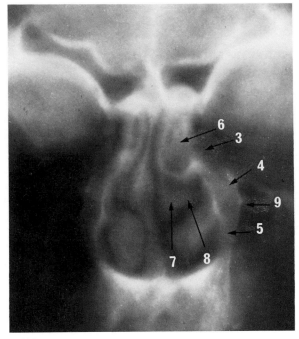

389b

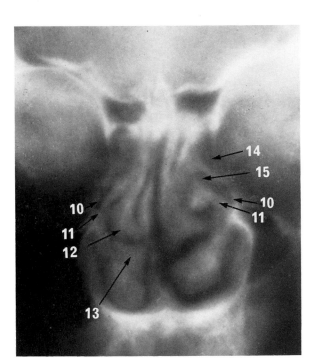

389c

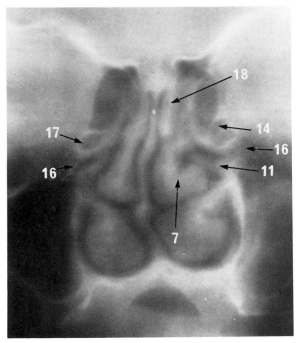

389d

389 a–d Tomograms of the anterior ethmoids, frontal sections, anterior to posterior, 5 mm apart

1 Tuberculum septi
2 Agger nasi cell
3 Lacrimal fossa
4 Lacrimal canal
5 Opening of lacrimal duct
6 Frontal recess
7 Concha sinus
8 Horizontal bony crest of the middle turbinate narrowing the middle meatus
9 Lacrimal prominence
10 Infundibulum
11 Medial wall of the infundibulum, projecting medially to form a double middle turbinate
12 Abnormally curved middle turbinate, narrowing the anterior middle meatus
13 Duplication of the inferior turbinate
14 Ethmoid bulla
15 Hiatus semilunaris
16 Maxillary sinus ostium
17 Anterior ethmoidal cell
18 Superior turbinate

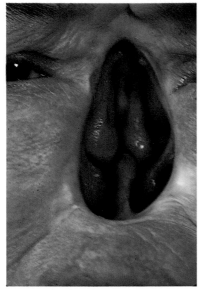

390

390 Interior of the nasal cavity
Complete destruction of the nasal pyramid and of the anterior septum following tertiary syphilis offers an unobstructed view of the inferior and middle turbinates on either side of the middle vomerian remnant below and the perpendicular plate of the ethmoid above.

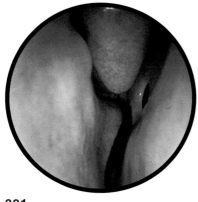

391

391 Maxillary sinus accessory ostium, endoscopic view
The ostium lies in the middle meatus between the middle and inferior turbinates. The nasal septum with a small spur is on the left of the photo.

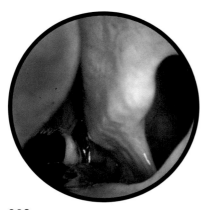

392

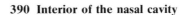

392a

392 Abnormally large natural ostium, maxillary sinus, left
It is possible to inspect the maxillary sinus with an angled telescope when the natural ostium is this large.

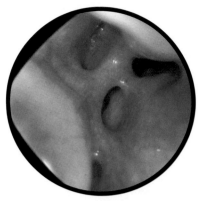

393

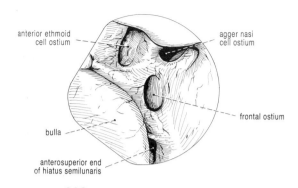

anterior ethmoid cell ostium

agger nasi cell ostium

frontal ostium

bulla

anterosuperior end of hiatus semilunaris

393a

393 View of the frontal recess, left
Lying in the anterior portion of the middle meatus, the frontal recess is a variable space associated with the anterior ethmoids and the frontal sinus. – In this photo the upper end of the hiatus semilunaris lies at 6 o'clock, limited superiorly by a bridge between the uncinate process

and the ethmoid bulla. Lateral to this bridge the infundibulum leads superiorly to the skull base. The frontal sinus ostium lies above this bridge. Adjacent to the frontal ostium there is an ostium of an agger nasi cell and, superiorly, another ostium of an anterior ethmoidal cell.

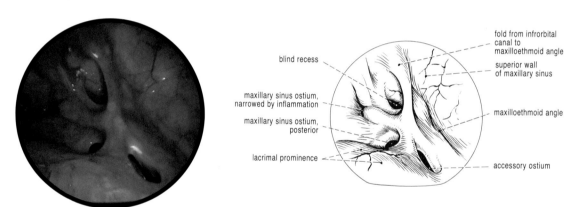

blind recess

maxillary sinus ostium, narrowed by inflammation

maxillary sinus ostium, posterior

lacrimal prominence

fold from infrorbital canal to maxilloethmoid angle

superior wall of maxillary sinus

maxilloethmoid angle

accessory ostium

394

394a

394 Ostia of the left maxillary sinus, intrasinus view
One or two ostia of the maxillary sinus usually open into the infundibulum. Accessory ostia can be noted in the inferior or posterior portion of the membranous wall of the sinus. At times a blind recess can extend towards the ethmoids. In this photograph, two ostia open into the infundibulum. The anterior ostium at 10 o'clock is nar-

rowed by mucosal edema. The posterior ostium lies just anterior to a fold which passes from the infraorbital canal to the maxillary-ethmoid angle. At 12 o'clock there is a blind-ended recess directed toward the ethmoids. There is an accessory oval ostium in the posterior membranous wall of the sinus at 5 o'clock.

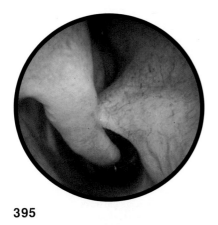

395

395 Septal spur, right
The spur is in contact with the inferior turbinate and obstructs nasal breathing and mucous drainage.

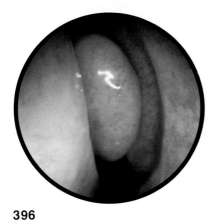

396

396 Enlarged ethmoid bulla, left
The enlarged bulla projects into the middle meatus. This finding can be an anatomical variant. An enlarged bulla,

396a

however, can fill the middle meatus, project onto the medial wall of the infundibulum, and narrow this area to cause infection of the sinuses.

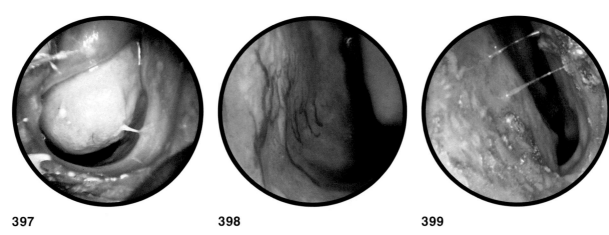

397   **398**   **399**

397 Encephalocele nasal cavity, right
The encephalocele arose from the roof of the nasal fossa in a ten-year-old. The whitish mass pulsated slightly and swelled with increased intracranial pressure with straining. The septum is to the right.

398 Kiesselbach triangle, left
There is an arterial plexus in the anteroinferior portion of the nasal septum. This plexus is the site of most epistaxis from various causes such as infection, manipulation, trauma, hypertension, and clotting defects.

399 Pigment deposition in the left vestibule of a dye worker

Trauma, Foreign Bodies, Infection

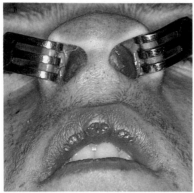

400

400 Infected septal hematoma
Two weeks earlier the patient suffered a blow to his nose. There was an epistaxis of short duration. He noted gradual increased difficulty in breathing through his nose and had a mild temperature elevation. The mucosa of both sides of the septum is so swollen that both nostrils are occluded.

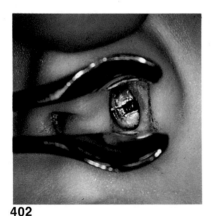

401

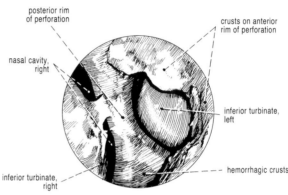

401a

401 Iatrogenic septal perforation
There are crusts at the margin of the septal perforation and compensatory hypertrophy of the turbinate. The perforation followed a submucous resection. The patient complained of frequent epistaxis, crusting, obstructed nasal breathing, and dryness in the nose.

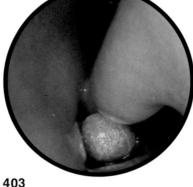 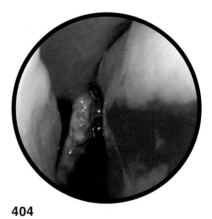

402   **403**   **404**

402–404 Intranasal foreign bodies
In Fig. **402** there is a metal screw in the left nostril of a four-year-old. Most nasal foreign bodies are located in the anterior nares and can be easily seen with the nasal speculum and good illumination. – Fig. **403** shows a marble in the anterior portion of the left nostril of a child. – When a foreign body is located in the posterior nares for a period of time and becomes infected, the diagnosis of a foreign body may be confused with that of an infection. It is important to remember that in children a unilateral foul-smelling nasal discharge is diagnostic of a foreign body. In Fig. **404** there is a piece of a cardboard carton lodged in the posterior nares. This patient was treated for sinusitis with antibiotics for one month before telescopic examination revealed the foreign body which was removed endoscopically.

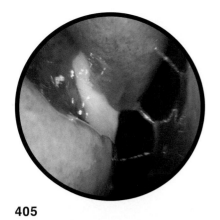

405

405 Acute purulent sinusitis, right
There is purulent secretion in the middle meatus with
edema of the uncinate process.

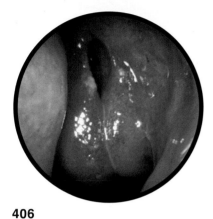

406

406 Doubled middle turbinate, left
This anatomical variant, a doubled middle turbinate, can
stenose the middle meatus and lead to obstruction of
drainage and infection of the maxillary and ethmoid
sinuses. In this patient, the edema and hyperplasia of the
mucosa of the affected middle turbinate are evidence of
repeated sinusitis.

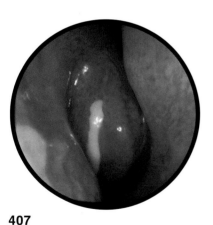

407

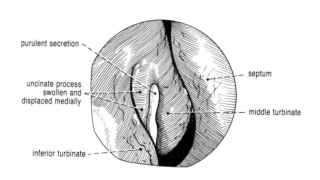

407 a

407 Ethmoid and maxillary sinus empyema, right
There is an empyema of the anterior ethmoid and maxillary sinuses. Purulent exudate flows from the narrowed
space between the middle turbinate and the edematous
infundibular wall.

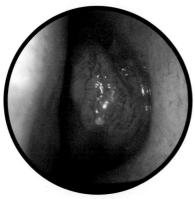

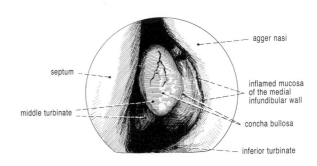

408

408a

408 Concha bullosa, left

A large infected cell in the anterior portion of the left middle turbinate obstructs drainage and ventilation of the anterior middle meatus. This infected cell has caused

an inflammation of the mucosa of the infundibulum. Endoscopic resection of the lateral portion of the turbinate and the infected cell relieved the stenosis and permitted the affected sinuses to heal.

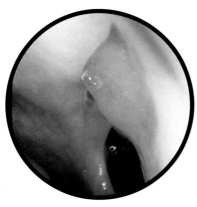

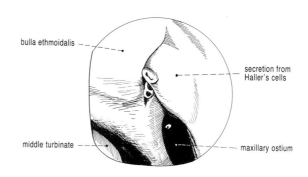

409

409a

409 Chronic ethmoiditis, left

Anterior ethmoid cells at times extend to the medial orbital floor and drain anterior and superior to the maxillary ostium below the bulla. Such cells are called Haller's cells in the German literature. This patient had radical maxillary sinus surgery several years previous to de-

veloping a purulent left nasal discharge. – The endoscopic view shows the discharge from infected Haller's cells. The purulence exudes above the maxillary ostium and below the bulla ethmoidalis. Following surgery of the affected ethmoid cells, the sinusitis cleared.

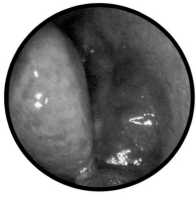

410

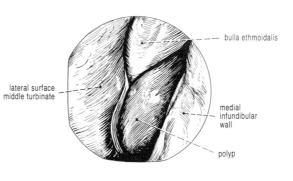

410a

410 Infected infundibulum, left
The infundibulum in the middle meatus opens into the semilunar hiatus. The variable-sized maxillary sinus ostium lies in the narrow space of the infundibulum floor. Anterior ethmoid cells also open into the infundibulum. The infundibulum can extend into the frontal recess and may extend laterally to the base of the skull. Fig. **410**

shows the endoscopic view of an abnormal infundibulum. The medial wall is edematous and enlarged medially to narrow the middle meatus. This finding can be the cause of recurrent maxillary and ethmoid sinusitis. Endoscopic resection of the medial infundibular wall will relieve the recurrent infections.

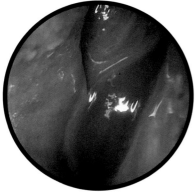
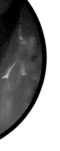

411

411a

411 Acute infection of the infundibulum, left
In this endoscopic view of the middle meatus, an edematous mucosal polyp from the infundibulum pro-

trudes into and obstructs the hiatus semilunaris between the bulla and the infundibular wall.

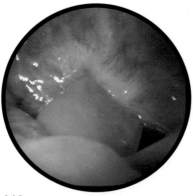

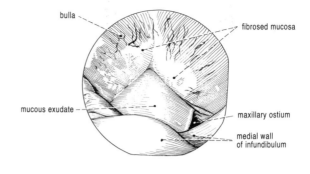

412

412a

412 Chronic infection of the infundibulum, left
This patient had two radical maxillary sinus procedures, but purulent exudate persisted. The endonasal view of the posterior half of the infundibulum shows viscid se-

cretion in the maxillary ostium. The mucosa of the ostium is edematous and scarred. Endoscopic resection of the infundibular wall relieved the condition.

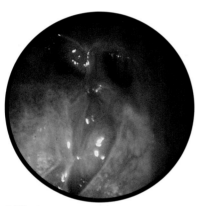

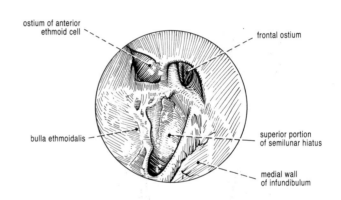

413

413a

413 Infected frontal recess, chronic frontal and ethmoid sinusitis, left
There is chronic frontal and ethmoidal sinusitis with in-

fected mucosa filling the infundibulum. In the frontal recess the ethmoid and frontal ostia are obstructed by swollen mucosa.

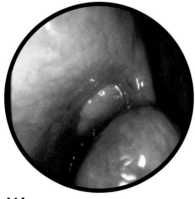

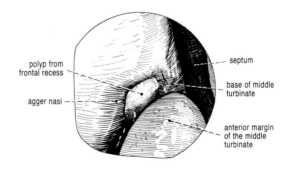

414

414a

414 Polypoid inflammation of the frontal recess, right
Following an acute rhinitis several weeks previously this patient developed obstructed nasal breathing and morning headaches. The floor of the frontal sinus was tender to pressure. An x-ray showed clouding of the frontal and

anterior ethmoid sinuses. The endoscopic view shows an edematous polyp from the frontal recess in the anterior portion of the middle meatus. An endoscopic removal of the polyp and medial wall of the infundibulum healed the sinusitis.

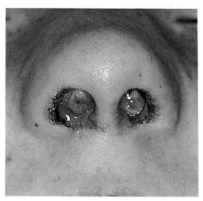

415

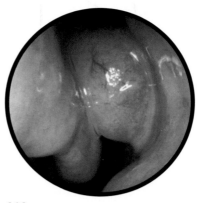

416

415 Obstructing nasal polyposis, bilateral
There was an associated chronic bilateral suppurative polyposis of the maxillary and ethmoid sinuses. Radiographs showed homogenous densities in the affected sinuses.

416 Solitary nasal polyp, right
This 58-year-old patient noted unilateral nasal obstruction. There is a single polyp arising from the lateral surface of the middle turbinate. The nasal septum is on the right.

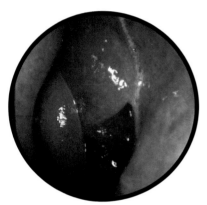

417

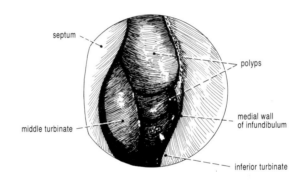

417a

417 Ethmoid polyposis
In this endoscopic view the polyps fill and occlude the left middle meatus. The findings on the right side were

identical. The nasal secretion and histology showed many eosinophils, and allergy tests were positive.

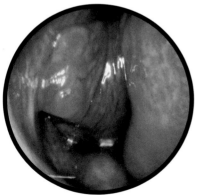

418

418 Allergic rhinitis, right
There is serous edema and swelling of the inferior turbinate in this 26-year-old hay fever victim.

Blow-out Fractures

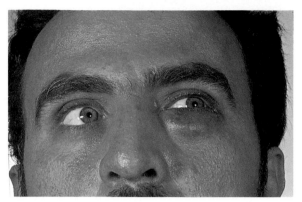

419

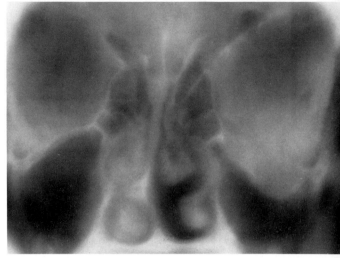

420

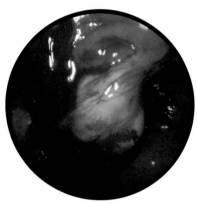

421

419–421 Blow-out fracture, left
This blow-out fracture, Fig. **419,** of the floor of the left orbit followed a fist blow to the eye. There are edema and subcutaneous emphysema of the infraorbital region, enophthalmos, paresthesia of the infraorbital nerve, and entrapment of the inferior oblique muscle with double vision. – Tomography, Fig. **420,** shows the bony defect of the orbital floor and the prolapsed soft tissue shadow of the orbital soft tissue in the maxillary sinus. – Sinoscopy, Fig. **421,** shows the soft tissue and the inferior oblique muscle caught in the herniation. The sinus mucosa is hemorrhagic.

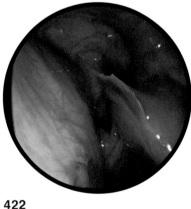

422

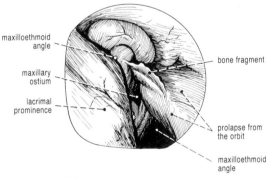

maxilloethmoid angle

maxillary ostium

lacrimal prominence

bone fragment

prolapse from the orbit

maxilloethmoid angle

422a

422 Blow-out fracture, sinoscopy, left
Following injury to the left eye by a tennis ball there is prolapse of orbital soft tissue into the sinus lumen. A bone fragment lies near the sinus ostium.

Acute and Chronic Sinusitis

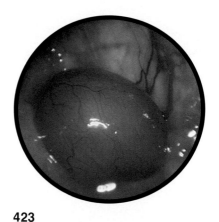

423

**423 Alveolar recess cyst, maxillary sinus, left, sinos-
copy**
This lesion was noted on an x-ray, but the patient had no
symptoms, and a dental work-up ruled out a dentigerous
cyst.

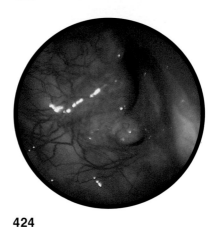

424

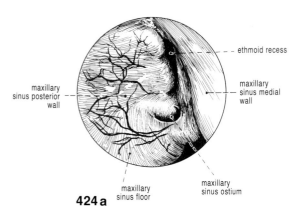

424 a

424 Acute maxillary sinusitis, sinoscopy, right
The mucosa of the medial sinus wall in the maxillo-ethmoid angle is injected and slightly edematous.

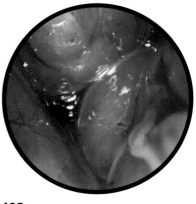

425

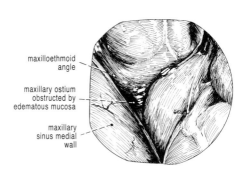

425 a

425 Chronic maxillary sinusitis, sinoscopy, left
This view shows chronic edematous infiltration and
broad-based polypoid degeneration of the mucosa of the
maxillo-ethmoidal portion of the sinus. The sinus ostium

is obstructed by marked mucosal thickening. The edema
and swelling around the ostium suggest involvement of
the infundibulum. The findings are similiar to those of an
allergic rhinosinusitis.

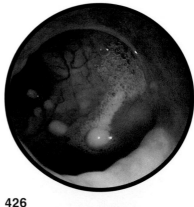

426

426 Chronic cystic maxillary sinusitis, right, endonasal view

The telescope shows a view through a large accessory maxillary sinus ostium in the midportion of the nasal cavity into the pterygoid recess of the antrum. Seen through the ostium there is an irregular nodular edema of the sinus mucosa from ectatic secretion-laden mucous glands.

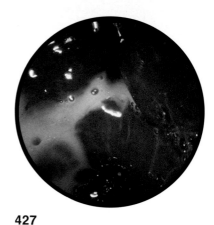

427

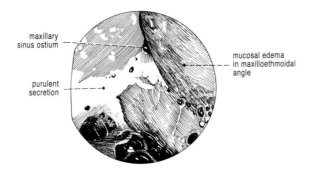

427 a

427 Empyema of the maxillary sinus, right, sinoscopy
Following puncture, pus under pressure flowed from this sinus. This is a view of the maxillo-ethmoid angle. There is a wide band of mucopurulent exudate leading to the

obstructed ostium. The mucosa is severely affected by edema and inflammation, which obstructs the ostium. Sinus lavage in cases such as this is difficult.

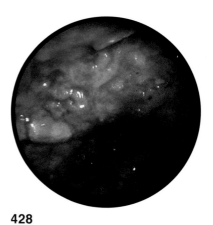

428

428 Chronic maxillary sinusitis, left, sinoscopy
X-ray showed thickening of the mucosa of the left maxillary sinus. Several irrigations of the sinus produced fetid pus. Sinoscopy shows nodular gray-white mucosa resembling a fungus infection. Biopsy showed extensive epithelial metaplasia resembling cholesteatoma matrix.

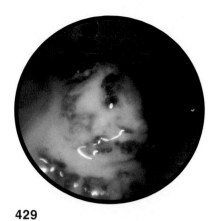

429

429 Mycosis maxillary sinus, left, sinoscopy
The patient had a chronic maxillary sinusitis resistant to therapy. Sinoscopy shows a yellow-brown concretion with black, irregular markings covered with purulent secretion. The cause of this concretion was an infection with Aspergillus niger.

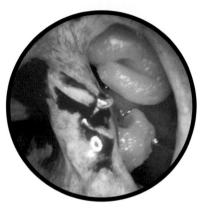

430

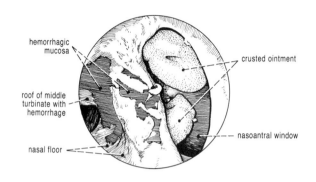

430a

hemorrhagic
mucosa

roof of middle
turbinate with
hemorrhage

nasal floor

crusted ointment

nasoantral window

430 Foreign body, ointment, maxillary sinus, left endonasal view
There is a mass of crusted ointment within the maxillary sinus seen through an antral window. The patient said that the ointment had been instilled as local therapy in his sinus through a nasoantral window 18 months previously.

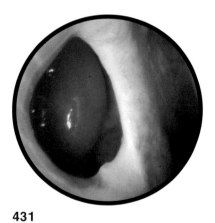

431

431 Residual polyp maxillary sinus, right endonasal view
There were continued symptoms following a maxillary sinus operation. This endonasal view through a large antral window in the inferior meatus shows a large residual polyp.

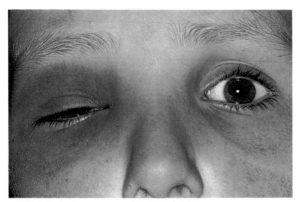

432

**432 Beginning orbital phlegmon from acute pan-
    sinusitis, right**
There is periorbital edema and erythema in this 11-
year-old girl caused by a right pansinusitis.

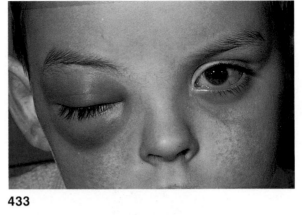

433

433 Suppurative orbital phlegmon, right
An orbital abscess is forming, and there are exophthalmos and chemosis. The nine-year-old patient has a suppurative right ethmoid and maxillary sinusitis which has
spread to the orbit.

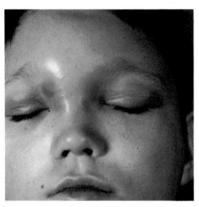

434

**434 Frontal sinusitis and osteomyelitis of the frontal
    bone**

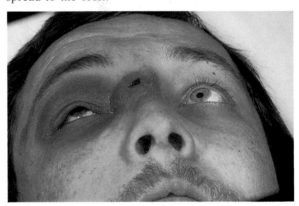

435

435 Infected sebaceous cyst, nasal roof, right
There is spread of infection to both lids.

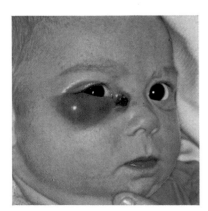

436

436 Superior maxillary osteomyelitis, right
The infant is 3 1/2 months old, and the lesion could have
arisen from a toothbud, the lacrimal sac or the ethmoids.

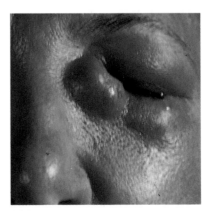

437

437 Lacrimal sac infection, left
There is an acute exacerbation of a chronic dacryocys-
titis with cellulitis of the surrounding tissue in this 48-
year-old patient.

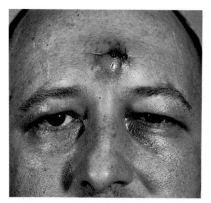

438

438 Pyocele left frontal sinus with fistula
The patient noted swelling of the forehead to the left of the midline for seven months. The family physician incised what appeared to be an infected sebaceous cyst, but pus continued to drain from the incision. The left palpebral fissure is narrowed. Radiographically, the floor of the frontal sinus and the medial orbital rim were destroyed by pressure atrophy of the lesion.

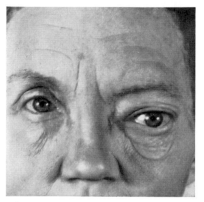

439

439 Frontal sinus pyomucocele, left
This 61-year-old female had external frontal sinus surgery 25 years previously. For the past six months she noted a swelling over the left eye with displacement of the orbit laterally and downward, and diplopia. This is a draining fistula in the old scar on the upper lid at the medial canthus.

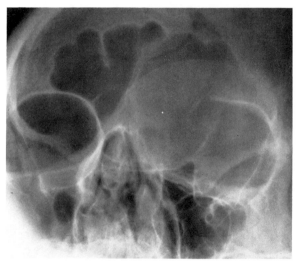

440

440 Pyomucocele, frontoethmoidal
The x-ray of another patient with a mucocele without previous surgery, but a similar clinical picture. There is homogeneous clouding of the frontal and ethmoid sinuses, and partial destruction of the bony floor of the frontal sinus and the adjacent orbital wall caused by the pressure of the pyomucocele.

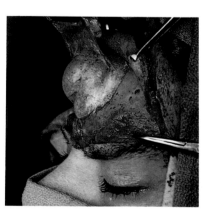

441

441 Bilateral frontal mucocele, surgical findings
This 24-year-old patient had clinical and radiographic findings of chronic pansinusitis with profuse intranasal polyps. For the past six months increased swelling of the anterior wall of the frontal sinus occurred. The photo shows the surgical exposure of the larger left mucocele.

Uncommon Diseases

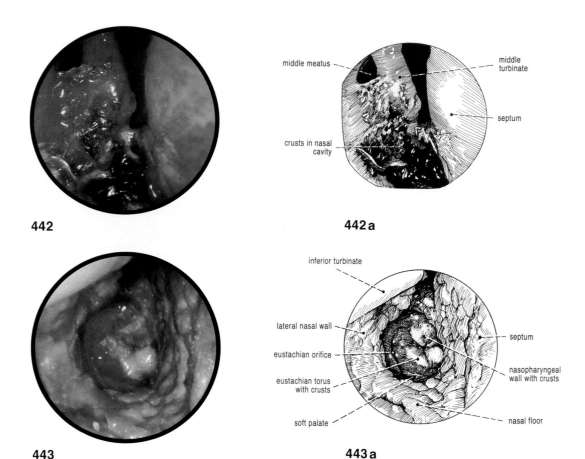

442

442a

443

443a

442–443 Ozena of the nose and nasopharynx
In Fig. **442** there is fetid crust formation in the entire right nostril and atrophy of the middle turbinate. – Fig. **443** shows the atrophic mucosa of the septum, the right nasal floor and the lateral nasal wall covered with over-lying yellow-green crusts. The nasal cavity is enlarged and the eustachian tube ostium and the crusted posterior nasopharynx wall are visible. The patient and his nearby neighbors could note the foul smell eminating from the nose.

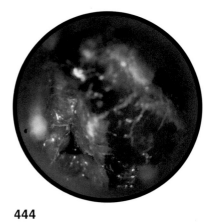

444

444 Lepromatous leprosy, endonasal findings, right
As is often the case with early involvement of the nasal mucosa in leprosy, this patient complained of recurrent epistaxis and nasal obstruction. Both nostrils were scarred, crusted, and narrowed. The narrowed nasal lumen lies inferiorly. This is the same patient as in Figs **38, 846.**

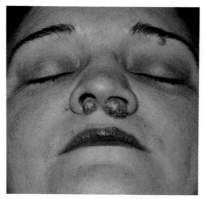

445

445 Rhinoscleroma

A 46-year-old female had a sixteen-year history of a nasal growth, which was histologically diagnosed as rhinoscleroma five years after its onset. The presence of K. *pneumoniae,* Type C or 3, confirmed the diagnosis. The nose is dilated and red, granular lesions fill both nares. A long course of antibacterial therapy rendered the lesion sterile, permitting surgical removal with no evidence of disease after a thirteen-year follow-up.

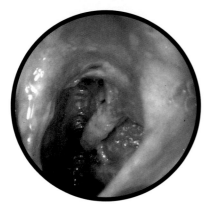

446

rhinoscleroma
scar in
nasal roof

septum

nasal lumen

middle turbinate

inferior turbinate

446a

446 Rhinoscleroma

An angled telescopic view from the oropharynx into the nasopharynx, through the choana, shows a long-standing rhinoscleroma with extensive atrophy and scarring on the left side. The olfactory portion of the nasal fossa is obstructed by scar tissue, and there is marked atrophy of the middle turbinate.

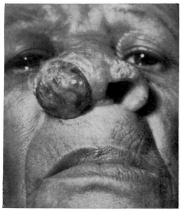

447

447 South American skin and mucous membrane leishmaniasis

A leishmaniasis-infiltrated polyp arises from the nasal septum and protrudes into the right nostril. There is mucosal ulceration of the left side of the septum and leishmanoid infiltration of the skin of the anterior external nose. See Figs **316, 317.**

Tumors

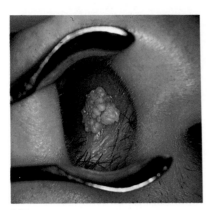

448

448 Benign papilloma of the septum
Papillomas have a predilection for the mucocutaneous junction of the nasal septum.

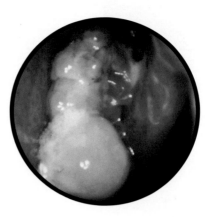

449

449 Inverting papilloma of the nose, left
A large tumor mass filling the middle meatus extends over the inferior turbinate and projects into the nasal cavity. Malignant degeneration of this lesion is not uncommon.

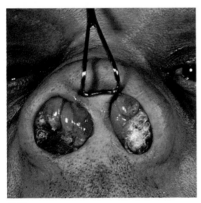

450

450 Inverting papilloma
This 53-year-old patient had multiple polypectomies over the past twenty years for recurrent nasal obstruction. He ultimately developed this extensive inverting papilloma which fills both nasal cavities, replaces the septum, and extends into both maxillary sinuses and the nasopharynx. The growth potential and the tendency for recurrence require radical surgical extirpation.

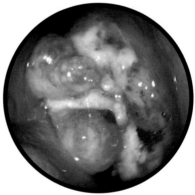

451

451 Transition of inverting papilloma to squamous cell carcinoma of the nose
Fig. **451** shows the endoscopic view of an inverting papilloma with transition into a squamous cell carcinoma. The patient is 74 years old and noted left nasal obstruction for several months, followed by a bloody purulent discharge of several weeks duration.

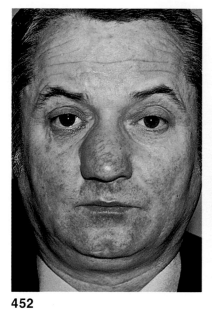

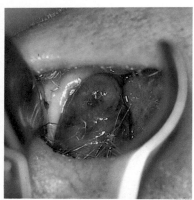

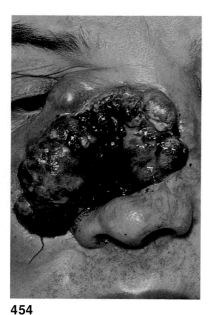

452   **453**   **454**

452–454 Malignant melanoma of the nose
Fig. **452** This 55-year-old male with a malignant melanoma of the nose noted nasal obstruction, epistaxis, and swelling of the right side of the nose. Fig. **453** shows the right nasal cavity obstructed by a malignant melanoma arising from the inferior turbinate. Im-

munologic and radiotherapy were ineffective. – Fig. **454:** External nose of the patient in Figs **452** and **453** seven months later. There has been an extremely rapid tumor growth with invasion of the sinuses, external extension, and diffuse metastases. The patient died shortly after.

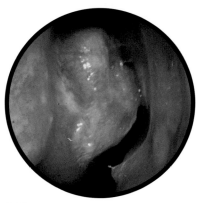

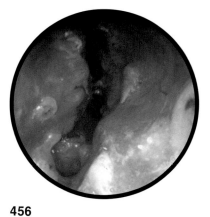

455   **456**

455 Squamous cell carcinoma of the nose
There is an ulcerated squamous cell carcinoma on the anterior portion of the inferior turbinate in a 26-year-old female. The main symptom was recurrent nasal bleeding.

456 Sarcoidosis of the nose
The chief symptoms of this patient were nasal bleeding, obstruction, and discharge. There is a granular lesion of the mucosa of the inferior turbinate and nasal floor. Such suspicious proliferating lesions always should be biopsied. Tuberculosis was suspected, but biopsy proved the lesion to be sarcoidosis.

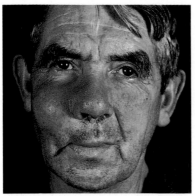

457

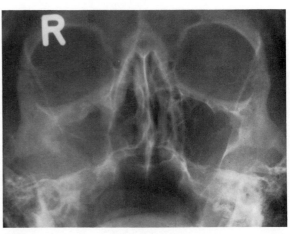

458

457–458 Squamous cell carcinoma of the maxillary sinus, right

The patient noted unilateral nasal obstruction and painless swelling in the right cheek. Within the month prior to this photo, the skin over the cheek swelled and became red. – Fig. **458** shows the x-ray findings. There is diffuse clouding and destruction of the bone of the lateral wall and floor of the antrum.

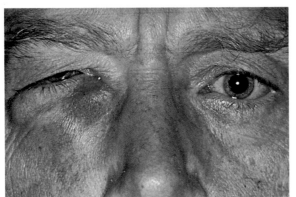

459

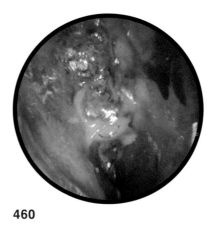

460

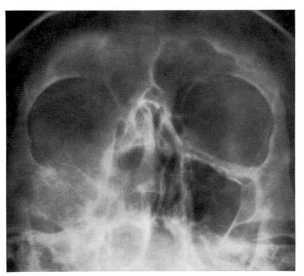

461

459–461 Squamous cell carcinoma of the maxillary and ethmoid sinuses, right

For several months this patient had pain in the right eye, nasal discharge, loss of smell, and tearing. The patient noted double vision and displacement of his right eye which caused him to seek medical advice, Fig. **459.** – In Fig. **460** the endonasal telescopic view shows tumor in the ethmoid region which was biopsied and showed malignancy. The x-ray, Fig. **461,** shows bony destruction of the medial and lateral walls of the maxillary sinus, the ethmoid sinuses and the orbital floor.

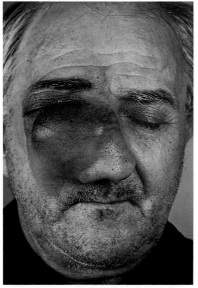

462

462 Extensive carcinoma of the maxillary sinus, right
There is massive involvement of the maxillary sinus, extending anteriorly and superiorly to the midportion of the face and orbit. Biopsy showed a squamous cell carcinoma. For precise diagnosis and staging of nasal cavity and paranasal sinus tumors endoscopy of the nose, paranasal sinuses and nasopharynx, tomography and biopsy are necessary.

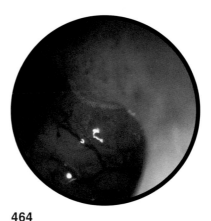

464

463–468 Adenoid cystic carcinoma
Adenoid cystic carcinomas generally are slow-growing lesions which originate in the major and minor salivary glands, and in the mucosa of the upper air and food passages, see Figs **346–351**. – The following photos, however, show an example of a fulmination course of this lesion over a period of 11 months. – This patient was a 38-year-old female. Symptoms began with leftsided facial pain and marked nasal obstruction. Examination showed a slight swelling of the left cheek and elevation of the eye, Fig. **463**. Intranasal, telescopic examination showed obstruction of the left nasal cavity by a vascular

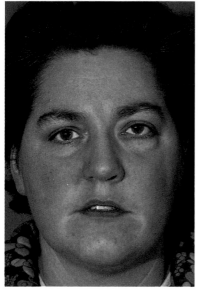

463

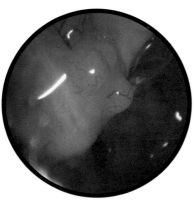

465

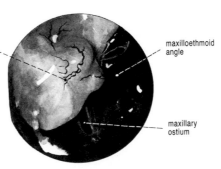

adenocystic carcinoma
infiltrating medial
antral wall

maxilloethmoid
angle

maxillary
ostium

465a

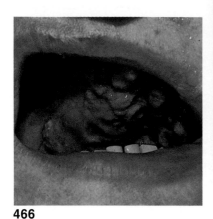

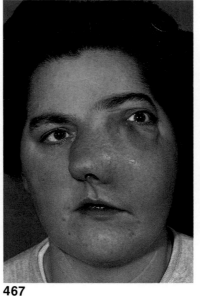

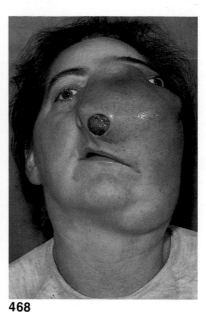

466

467

468

polypoid tumor mass, Fig. **464.** Endoscopic examination of the left maxillary sinus showed nodular infiltrating tumor involving the lacrimal prominence on the medial wall of the sinus, Fig. **465.** – Three months later, the tumor had involved the oral vestibule, the alveolar ridge and palate, Fig. **466.** At this time a chest x-ray showed lung metastases. – Figs **467** and **468** show further rapid progression of this lesion over a period of a few weeks. There were submaxillary lymph node metastases and destruction of the bone of the maxillary sinus and displacement of the eye due to orbital extension.

Diseases of the Nasopharynx and Choanae

Clinical Anatomy

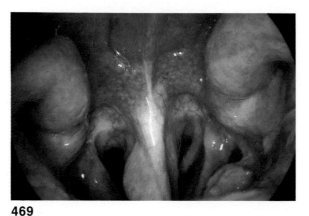

469

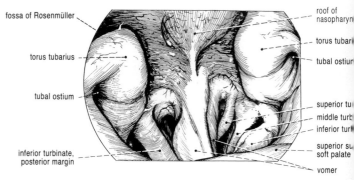

469a

fossa of Rosenmüller

torus tubarius

tubal ostium

inferior turbinate,
posterior margin

roof of
nasopharyn

torus tubari

tubal ostiur

superior tu
middle turb
inferior tur
superior su
soft palate

vomer

469 90°-telescopic view of the normal nasopharynx exposes both eustachian tube ostia, the choanae and roof of the nasopharynx.

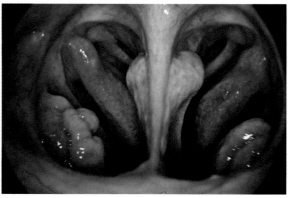

470

470 Choanae
The posterior extremities of the turbinates are visible. There are discrete mulberry swellings at the posterior margins of both inferior turbinates and mucosal cushions on both sides of the vomer.

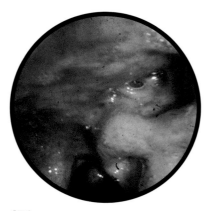

471

471 Rosenmüller's fossa, right
The choana, posterior end of the middle turbinate and vomer are visible.

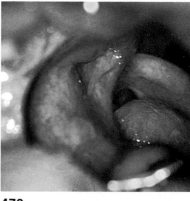

472

472 Choana and eustachian tube orifice, right
This photo shows the tubal orifice as seen with the nasopharyngeal mirror. The posterior ends of the middle and inferior turbinates are also visualized.

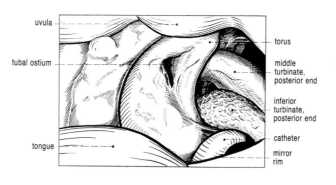

472a

uvula

tubal ostium

tongue

torus

middle
turbinate,
posterior end

inferior
turbinate,
posterior end

catheter

mirror
rim

Congenital Anomalies

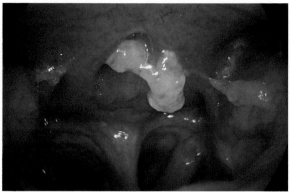

473

473 Nasopharynx, Rathke's pouch
There is thick secretion in the pouch lumen.

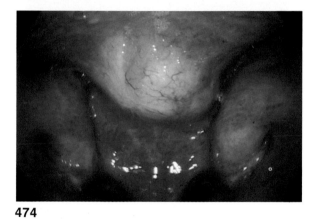

474

474 Nasopharynx, Thornwaldt's cyst
The cyst lies on the nasopharyngeal roof. The tubal ostia lie laterally.

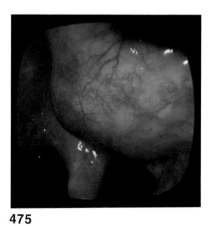

475

475 Meningoencephalocele, nasopharynx
There is a large meningoencephalocele arising from the roof of the nasopharynx. The mass pulsates, and when the patient performs the Valsalva maneuver the mass enlarges. In lesions such as this, neurologic consultation and CT scanning are indicated. This type of lesion should be biopsied only after extensive work-up and with great care.

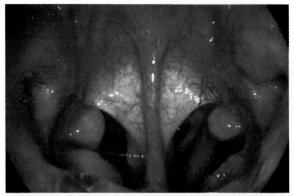

476

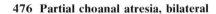
476 Partial choanal atresia, bilateral

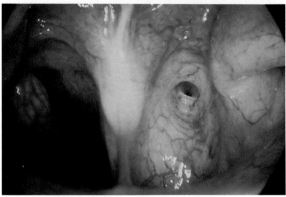

477

477 Choanal atresia membranous, unilateral, right
The right choana is completely occluded in this 18-
year-old male who noted lifelong unilateral nasal obstruction. There is a minute retracted, blind pit in the
membrane closing the choana. The left choana is patent.

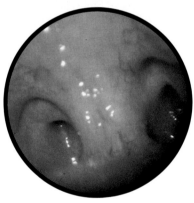

478

478 Choanal atresia, bony, bilateral
There is a bilateral bony atresia in this three-week-old
infant. Infants with bilateral choanal atresia have severe
respiratory and sucking difficulties. The posterior end of
the vomer is abnormally widened.

Hyperplasia and Inflammation

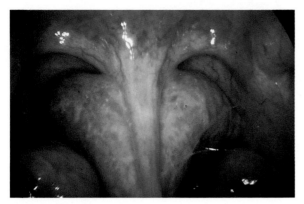

479

479 Vomer cushions, bilateral
This 58-year-old male noted partial nasal obstruction for many years.

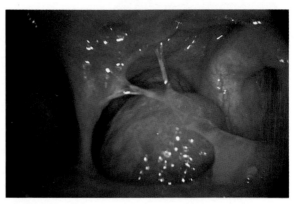

480

480 Enlargement of posterior end of inferior turbinate, right
The right choana is almost completely obstructed by hypertrophy of the posterior end of the inferior turbinate. Note the mucous strands overlying the hypertrophic area.

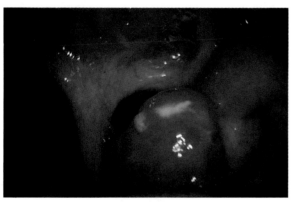

481

481 Choanal polyp, right
The polyp arises from the maxillary sinus ostium. The patient complained of right cheek pain and unilateral obstructed nasal breathing, and x-ray of the right antrum showed clouding (90°-telescopic view).

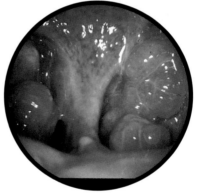

482

482 Choanal polyps, bilateral
This patient had polyps filling both nostrils, chronic bilateral polypoid sinusitis, and chronic bronchitis. He complained of chronic bilateral nasal discharge and obstruction.

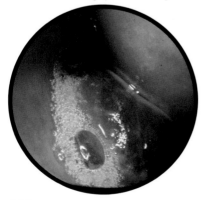

483

483 Choanal polyp, transnasal view, right

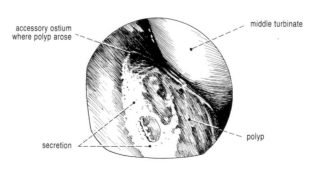

483a

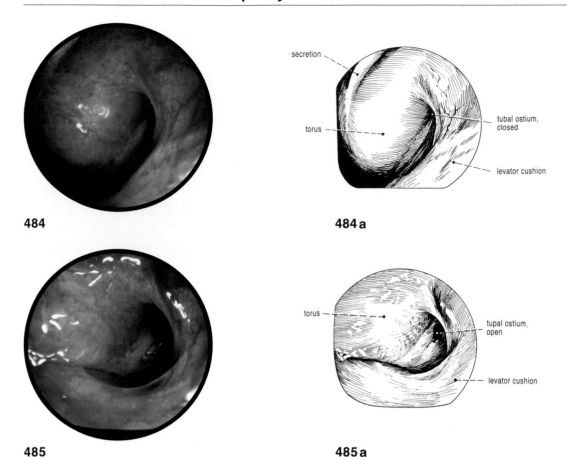

484

484a

485

485a

484–485 Eustachian tube at rest and during swallowing, left

Fig. **484** shows the tube orifice at rest when it is normally closed. Fig. **485** was taken during swallowing and shows the opening of the tube (transnasal endoscopic view).

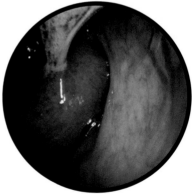

486

486 Hyperplasia, torus tubarius

Transnasal endoscopy shows that hyperplasia of the torus has caused narrowing of the tubal ostium. Thick nasal secretions stretch over the torus and the narrowed tubal ostium. There was a secretory otitis media on this side due to the chronic rhinitis.

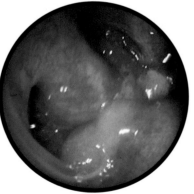

487

487 Nasopharyngeal mucopurulent secretion

The transnasal photo shows purulent secretion being forced into the ostium of the eustachian tube during swallowing.

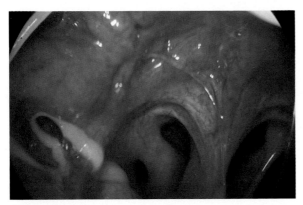

488

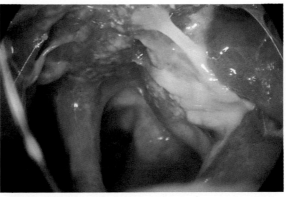

489

488 Mucopurulent discharge in the nasopharynx
There is a strand of mucopurulent discharge in the left choana which flows over the eustachian tube ostium. The secretion originated in a chronic infection of the left antrum in a 19-year-old male. The patient had a chronic left secretory otitis media.

489 Nasopharyngitis sicca, ozena
This 42-year-old female had chronic polyarthritis, and saw an otolaryngologist because of recurrent bilateral secretory otitis media. The examination shows crusted purulent secretion obstructing the right tubal ostium (s. Figs. **442–443, 688**).

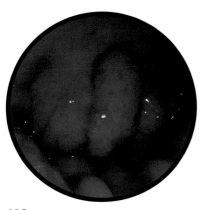

490

490 Hypertrophic adenoids
The hypertrophic, furrowed adenoids almost completely fill the nasopharynx and obstruct the choanae.

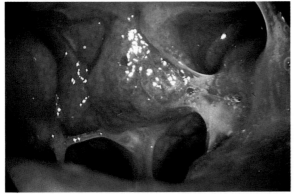

491

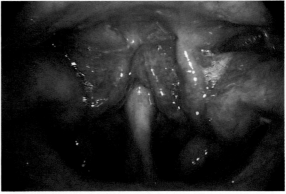

492

491 Minimal hypertrophy of the adenoids
There is mucopurulent discharge around the right eustachian tube ostium. The patient suffered from repeated attacks of acute otitis media.

492 Residual adenoid tissue on the torus tubarius
Following incomplete adenoidectomy or regrowth of lymphoid tissue, there is lymphoid hypertrophy on both toruses seen at 9 and 3 o'clock in the photo. This 15-year-old boy suffered recurrent episodes of secretory otitis media.

Tumors

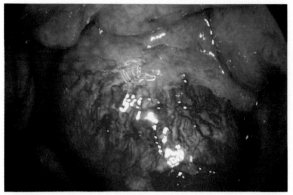

493

493 Juvenile hemangiofibroma of the nasopharynx
There is a large, globular, vascular tumor lying in the nasopharynx, partially obstructing both choanae. The tumor has a broad base located on the posterior wall of the nasopharynx. The eustachian tube orifices and lateral portion of the choanae are visible. The patient was a 14-year-old male who noted increasing nasal obstruction and recurrent epistaxis for several months before seeing his physician.

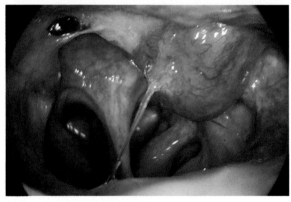

494

494 Lymphoepithelial carcinoma, nasopharynx
This 40-year-old male noted a right-sided hearing loss for a year prior to examination and photography. A swelling in the upper lateral portion of his neck brought him to a physician. Neck biopsy showed a lymphoepithelial carcinoma, the Schmincke tumor. He was then referred to the otolaryngologist to locate the primary lesion. The rounded, red lesion is visible endoscopically on the right side of the nasopharyngeal roof where it is infiltrating the right eustachian tubal orifice.

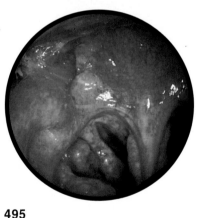

495   **495a**

495 Lymphoepithelial carcinoma, persistent
Despite a full course of 6000 rads of radiotherapy, there is residual tumor in the Fossa of Rosenmüller and the torus tubarius left. The slightly nodular lesion, partially covered by mucous extends toward the roof of the nasopharynx. Tumor infiltration of the torus caused a persistent secretory otitis and conductive deafness. The elevated Ebstein-Barr virus titer persisted after therapy.

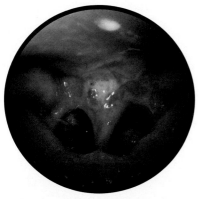

496

496 Squamous cell carcinoma, nasopharynx
The small ulcerated lesion lies in the midportion of the nasopharyngeal roof. There were no nasopharyngeal symptoms, but there were bilateral cervical lymph node metastases.

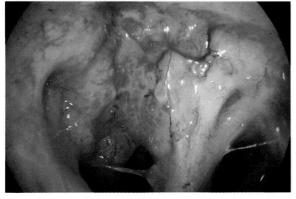

497

497 Squamous cell carcinoma, nasopharynx, left
The raised, granular tumor lies on the nasopharyngeal roof and extends to the torus tubarius in this 44-year-old male. The symptoms were unilateral secretory otitis and left cervical metastases.

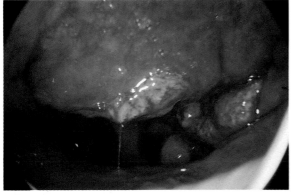

498

498 Squamous cell carcinoma, nasopharynx
This large, granular, ulcerated lesion of the nasopharynx has involved the left torus tubarius and extended across the midline to invade the right tubal ostium. The choanae are visible. Both tubal ostiums are obstructed.

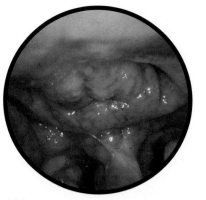

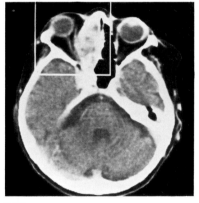

tumor in
nasopharyngeal
roof

left choana

right choana

septum

499

499a

499 Lymphocytic, non-Hodgkin's Lymphoma
According to the staging work-up by the internist and

the radiologist, the first manifestation of this malignant lymphoma was this mass in the nasopharynx.

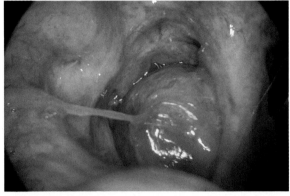

500

500 Plasmocytic lymphoma, posterior end of inferior turbinate, left
In the left choana there is a rounded tumor partially covered by yellow secretion on the posterior end of the inferior turbinate. This 73-year-old patient noted nasal obstruction on this side for one year. Biopsy showed a plasmocytic lymphoma. The vomer is at the right.

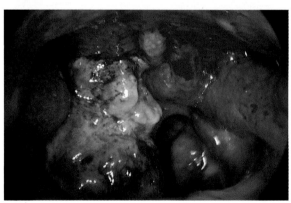

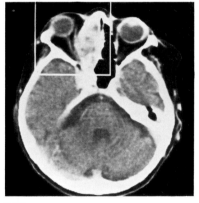

501

502

501–502 Rhabdomyosarcoma
For three months this 70-year-old male noted obstructed left nasal breathing and recurrent epistaxis. The entire left nasal cavity is filled with an easily bleeding tumor which extends to the nasopharynx. Within a few days the lesion caused left exophthalmos and double vision. Biopsy showed a rhabdomyosarcoma. – Fig. **501**

shows the extent of the lesion into the nasopharynx through the left choana. – Fig. **502** is the CT showing tumor invasion of the entire left nasal cavity and the adjacent paranasal sinuses with breakthrough into the orbit causing the exophthalmos. The extension into the nasopharynx is visible.

Diseases of the Oropharynx and the Hypopharynx

Diseases of the Oropharynx

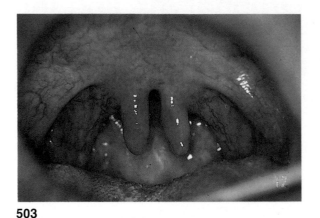

503

503 Bifida uvula

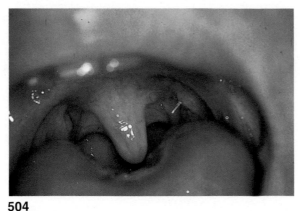

504

504 Foreign body, fish bone, tonsil, superior pole, left

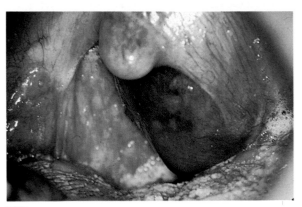

505

505 Branchiogenic cyst, oropharyngeal view, left
This 35-year-old man gave a history of a swelling in the left neck since infancy. Tonsillectomy and removal of a cyst from the left tonsil area had been performed at 5 years of age, and the cyst in the throat had been aspirated several times in the interim. During the previous two months the cyst had doubled in size and become painful, and the patient had experienced difficulty in swallowing. External surgical resection showed it to be multilocular, extending between the carotid bifurcation to its point of attachment behind the left posterior pillar.

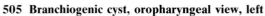

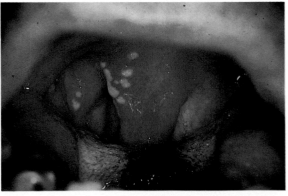

507

506

506 Chordoma, oropharynx, left
This 75-year-old male gave a history of progressive difficulty in swallowing for three years. A large mass filled the left oro- and nasopharynx, producing a palpable fullness of the mandibular and submandibular area. Chordomas are fetal rests of the chorda dorsalis arising usually from the clivus and extending into the nasopharynx, the sphenoid or adjacent sinuses. Depending on their location and extent, they may produce tubal and nasal blockage and even neurologic signs. Differing from histologically malignant tumors, they are covered by a smooth mucosa and are of long-standing duration.

507 Aphthous tonsillitis and uvulitis
There is an associated black hairy tongue.

Palatine Tonsils

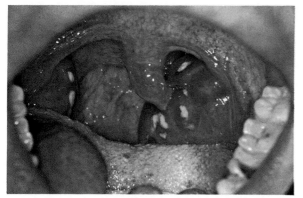

508

508 Acute follicular tonsillitis
There is left-sided tonsillar hypertrophy, and exudate fills the crypts of both tonsils. The patient noted pain on swallowing, and there were leucocytosis, elevated temperature, and painful swelling of the cervical lymph nodes.

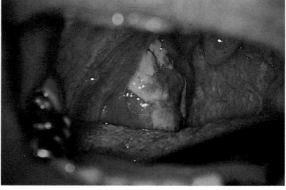

509

509 Exudative tonsillitis
This swollen right tonsil was covered by a thick exudate in a 47-year-old male who was found to have granulocytopenia related to Hodgkin's disease.

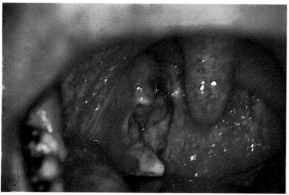

510

510 Plaut-Vincent's angina
This 21-year-old patient complained of slight pain on swallowing on the right side of his throat for the past week. The temperature was normal, and there was only a slight general malaise despite the marked ulceromembranous unilateral lesion of the right tonsil. In Plaut-Vincent's angina there frequently is a discrepancy be-

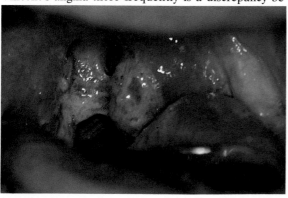

512

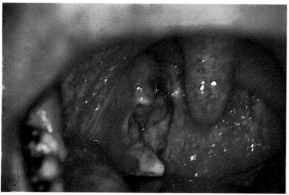

511

tween rather severe local findings and minimal systemic symptoms. A stained smear of the exudate showed the typical fusiform rods associated with the characteristic spirochetes, pathognomonic for Plaut-Vincent's angina. – The differential diagnosis of this unilateral lesion should rule out primary and secondary syphilis, tuberculosis, an ulcerated, necrotic carcinoma, leukemia, and agranulocytosis.

511 Pseudomembranous acute tonsillitis
In cases such as in this 24-year-old male, it is necessary to rule out mononucleosis (see Fig. **512**), diphtheria, and, rarely, pneumococcus as the causative agent. Pneumococcus was cultured in this patient.

512 Acute tonsillitis due to infectious mononucleosis
This 21-year-old male has marked bilateral cervical lymph node swelling and leucocytosis with increased mononucleocytes on the differential. The heterophil agglutination test was positive.

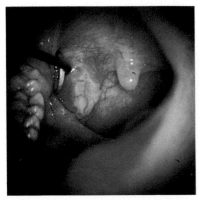

513

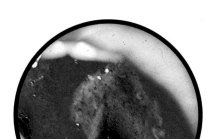

514

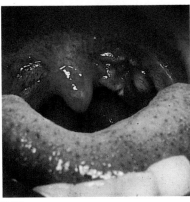

516

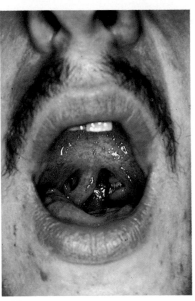

515

513 Tuberculosis of the tonsil
This infiltrative, ulcerated and membranous lesion of the right tonsil was associated with active lung tuberculosis. There is a superficial inflammation of the mucosa surrounding the tonsil.

514–516 Syphilis
Fig. **514** shows a primary luetic lesion of the left soft palate and uvula in a 21-year-old male. – Fig. **515** is a primary lesion in the left tonsil. Transition to a maculopapular exanthem of secondary syphilis is visible in the skin of the face. A primary syphilis lesion, as shown here, is frequently painful and firm to palpation. In this stage the lesion is highly infectious and the physician must wear rubber gloves when palpating such lesions. – Fig. **516** is an example of secondary luetic mucosal lesions. There are distinct opalescent plaques on the uvula and both tonsils. See Figs. **562–566,** and **598**.

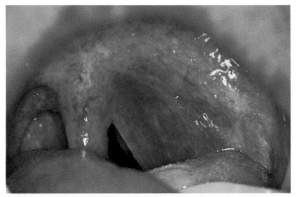

517

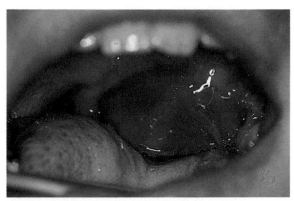

518

517–518 Peritonsillar abscess, left
Fig. **517** shows the early stage of a peritonsillar abscess. In spite of antibiotic therapy the condition worsened, there was trismus, distorted speech, leucocytosis, and fever. – Fig. **518** shows the full-blown picture of a peritonsillar abscess with the uvula displaced to the side opposite the abscess.

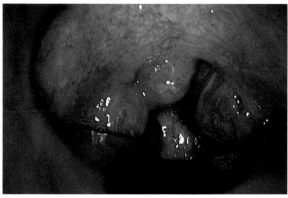

519

519 Chronic tonsillitis
This 18-year-old patient complained of recurrent mild pain on swallowing and a fetid breath. There is hypertrophy and swelling of both tonsils, and the anterior tonsillar pillars are reddened. A thin seropurulent secretion and necrotic debris exude from the crypts. There is mild bilateral cervical lymph node enlargement and tenderness.

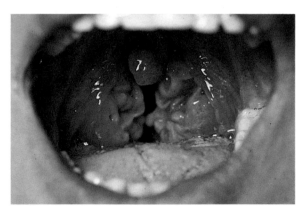

520

520 Hyperplastic tonsils

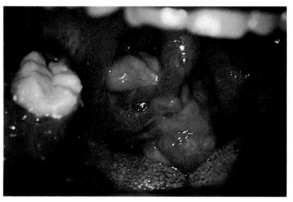

521

521 Chronic tonsillitis with unilateral hypertrophy, right
This 19-year-old patient complained of frequent sore throats and occasional swelling and pain in the neck. Unilateral tonsillar hypertrophy always requires a biopsy to rule out such lesions as lymphoma, carcinoma and pleomorphic adenoma. Histology of this tonsil following tonsillectomy showed chronic inflammation (s. Fig. **531**).

Tumors

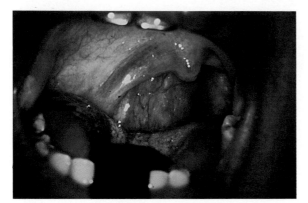

522

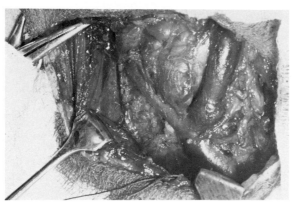

523

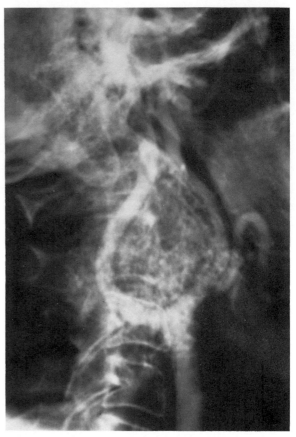

524

522–524 Carotid body tumor with pharyngeal involvement, right

This 32-year-old patient noted loud pulsating tinnitus and mild hearing loss for several years. There is a pulsating tumor mass in the right oropharynx, Fig. **522.** –

Carotid angiography, Fig. **524,** shows the characteristic widening of the angle of bifurcation of the external and internal carotid arteries by the large tumor mass. – Fig. **523** shows the carotid body tumor at surgery.

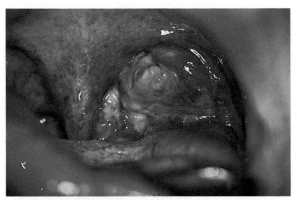

525

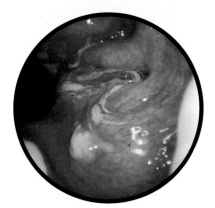

526

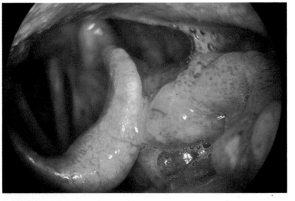

Rosenmüller's
fossa

torus

tubal ostium

soft palate

tumor infiltrating
the palate

526 a

**525–526 Squamous cell carcinoma, undifferentiated,
oropharynx, left**
This 71-year-old patient complained of left otalgia and
hearing loss for 4 weeks. There were cervical metastases.

Telescopic transnasal examination of the same patient
shows tumor infiltration of the levator palatini muscle
and partial obstruction of the left tubal ostium, Fig. **526.**

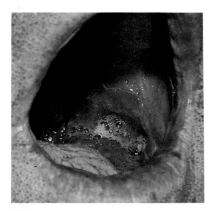

527

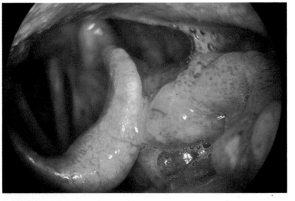

528

527–528 Squamous cell carcinoma of the tonsil
This extensive lesion, Fig. **527,** has spread to the soft
palate and the base of the tongue.

Fig. **528** is a 90°-telescopic view of the tumor spread in
the pharyngoepiglottic fold. There were large fixed cervical metastases and osteolysis of the mandible. The patient was a 71-year-old heavy smoker.

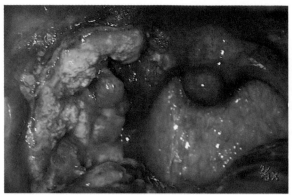

529

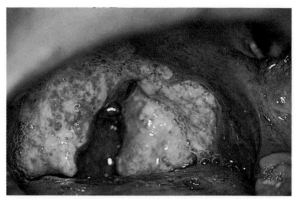

530

529 Squamous cell carcinoma oropharynx, right
There is an extensive, exophytic ulcerated carcinoma involving the tonsil, the soft palate, the lateral pharyngeal wall, and the base of the tongue. There are cervical metastases.

530 Squamous cell carcinoma, oropharynx
There is an ulcerative, membranous, papillary tumor involving both sides and posterior wall of the pharynx. The patient was 32 years old and a heavy smoker and drinker.

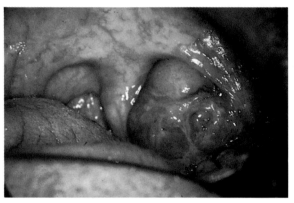

531

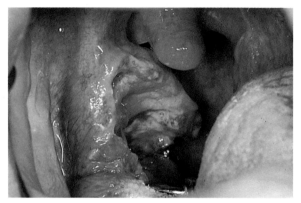

532

531 Immunoblastic lymphoma tonsil, left
The homolateral cervical lymph nodes were enlarged in this 70-year-old female. Staging showed no other evidence of dissemination beyond the cervical nodes.

532 Malignant lymphoma, oropharynx, right
Besides this ulcerated pharyngeal lesion in this 53-year-old male there was mediastinal lymph node enlargement, and nuclide studies showed involvement of the spleen.

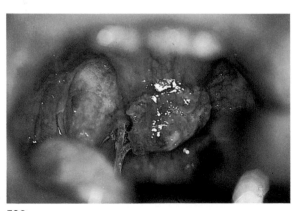

533

533 Squamous cell carcinoma of the uvula
This nodular lesion occurred in a 39-year-old chronic alcoholic who was a heavy smoker.

Base of Tongue and Vallecula

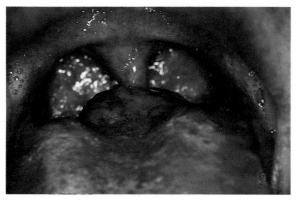

534

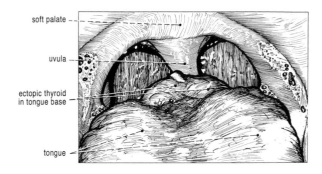

534 a

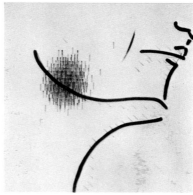

535

534–535 Ectopic thyroid gland, tongue base
Oral examination, Fig. **534,** shows a rounded, smooth tumor with vascular markings in the base of the tongue. – Fig. **535** is the radionuclide scan showing ectopic thyroid tissue in the tongue base. The patient was a 51-year-old hypothyroid female.

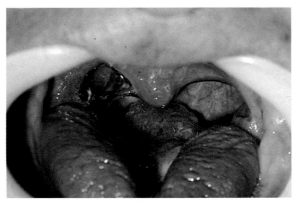

536

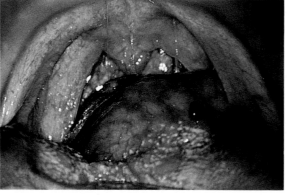

537

536 Squamous cell carcinoma of the epiglottis extending to the oropharynx
This 63-year-old male noted a sensation of fullness in his throat for one year and, recently, difficulty in swallowing. Depression of the tongue with a tongue blade exposes the large nodular tumor at the base of the tongue. There were bilateral fixed cervical metastases.

537 Carcinomatous degeneration of a pleomorphic adenoma in the base of the tongue
This 60-year-old patient gave a history similar to the patient in Fig. **536.** This lesion arose from the minor salivary glands of the tongue.

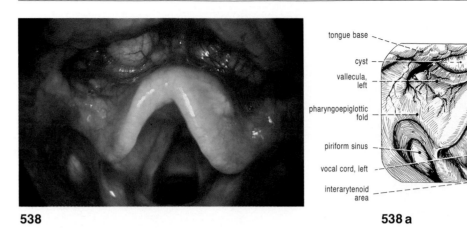

538

538a

Diagram labels (left side): tongue base, cyst, vallecula, left, pharyngoepiglottic fold, piriform sinus, vocal cord, left, interarytenoid area

Diagram labels (right side): glossoepiglottic fold, tongue base, vallecula, right, petiolus, pharyngoepiglottic fold, piriform sinus, epiglottis

538 Vallecular cyst, left
This is a fairly common and usually asymptomatic lesion, 90°-telescopic view.

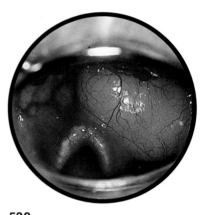

539

539 Vallecular cyst, left
This mucous retention cyst of the vallecula occurred in a nine-year-old boy. This child noted a sensation of a lump in his throat. Enlargement of such a cyst can lead to dysphonia, dyspnea, and even suffocation (mirror view).

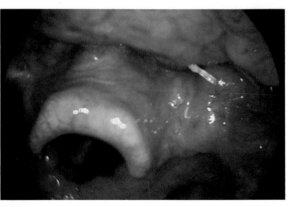

540

540 Foreign body, fish bone in the vallecula, right
The fish bone lies in the vallecula, and there is minimal mucosal edema. The patient felt a sticking sensation in his throat on swallowing. The 90°-telescope facilitated discovery of the bone.

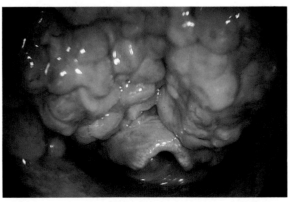

541

541 Hypertrophic lingual tonsil
Such marked hypertrophy causes symptoms of a lump in the throat, frequent clearing of the throat and dysphagia. A lymphoma or other malignancy must be ruled out by biopsy.

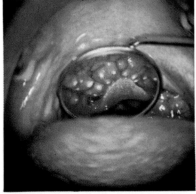

542

542 Lingual tonsillitis
A young adult female complained of an acute sore throat. The oropharynx was normal, but indirect examination with the mirror disclosed an acute inflammation of the lingual tonsil with exudate in many of the crypts.

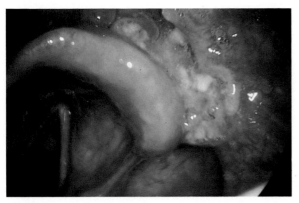

543

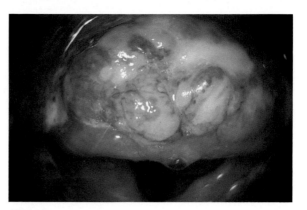

544

543 Squamous cell carcinoma of the vallecula, right
There is an exophytic, ulcerated lesion in the vallecula extending into the base of the tongue and lingual surface of the epiglottis. The patient was a 54-year-old alcoholic and heavy smoker. The tumor free larynx is seen in the photo at the left.

544 Adenoid cystic carcinoma of the lingual surface of the epiglottis
The lesion occurred in a 79-year-old nonsmoker. He complained of otalgia for six months. Difficulty in swallowing led the patient to see an otolaryngologist.

Diseases of the Hypopharynx

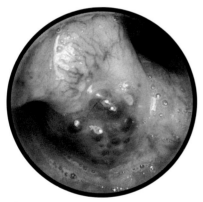

545

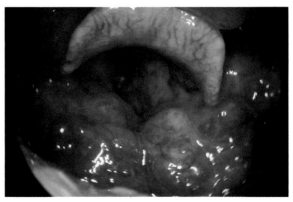

546

545 Cavernous hemangioma of the hypopharynx
A mulberry-like hemangioma, involving the left arytenoid and piriform sinus in a 43-year-old woman, is seen in the retrolaryngeal space. The patient described a vague discomfort and the sensation of a lump in the throat.

546 Hemangiomatosis of the larynx and hypopharynx
There is an extensive hemanigoma involving both piriform sinuses, the postcricoid region, the posterior wall of the hypopharynx, and the endolarynx. The patient saw an otolaryngologist for shortness of breath after having noted dysphagia for several months.

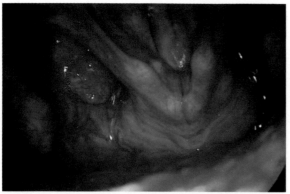

547

547 Squamous cell carcinoma of the piriform sinus, left
The first sign of this small, nodular broad-based lesion of the lateral wall of the piriform sinus was a lymph node metastasis. There is mucous medial to the tumor and in the opposite piriform sinus. Cervical lymph node metastases are frequently the first sign of piriform sinus malignancies.

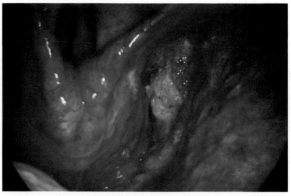

548

548 Squamous cell carcinoma of the piriform sinus, second primary, right
This 42-year-old construction worker, a heavy smoker and drinker, came to the otolaryngologist because of a squamous cell carcinoma of the alveolar ridge. He had worn dentures for six years. Examination of the pharynx revealed this asymptomatic, ulcerated second carcinoma on the lateral and anterior wall of the right piriform sinus. There were unilateral cervical metastases.

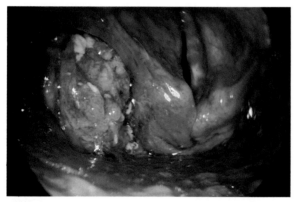

549

549 Squamous cell carcinoma of the hypopharynx, left
The left piriform sinus is filled with a nodular, ulcerated carcinoma. A long-standing dysphagia did not seem to bother the patient, but he sought medical attention because of increasing hoarseness and dyspnea. The tumor has infiltrated the left side of the larynx and metastasized fixed lymph nodes of the ipsilateral side.

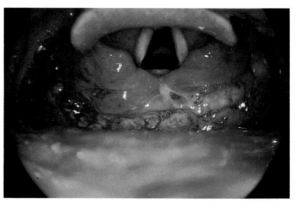

550

550 Squamous cell carcinoma of the postcricoid region
There is a circular, ulcerated carcinoma on the postcricoid area which extends onto the posterior hypopharyngeal wall and superior portion of the esophagus. The lesion bled spontaneously. The female patient was a 48-year-old Scandinavian nonsmoker who was treated for five years for the Plummer-Vinson syndrome.

Diseases
of the Mouth

**(Lips, Tongue, Oral Mucosa,
and Palate)**

Diseases of the Lips

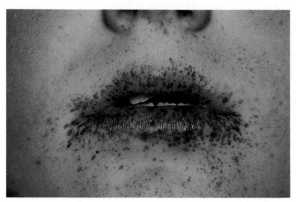

551

551 Peutz-Jeghers syndrome
There are perioral and labial speckled pigmentations as a result of a congenital malformation of the pigment cells. There often is intestinal polyposis associated with this congenital syndrome.

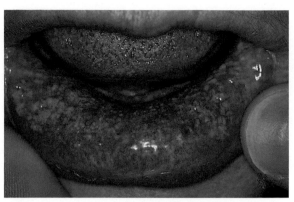

552

552 Amyloidosis of the lower lip mucosa, secondary to metastatic plasmacytoma of bone
This 62-year-old female has gelatinous macular deposits of amyloid in the translucent mucosa. There is marked dryness of the mouth.

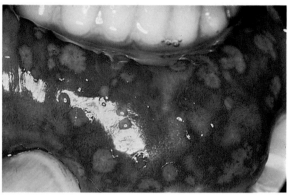

553

553 Herpes simplex of the mucosa of the lower lip

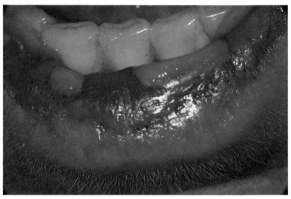

554

554 Pemphigus bullae of the lower lip

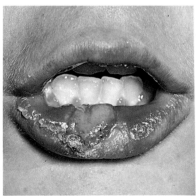

555

555 Pyostomatitis vegitans of the lip
This is a special form of chronic pyoderma (McCarthy) that rarely proliferates into the dermal portion of the lips. Occasionally this condition is associated with intestinal disturbances, such as colitis or ulcerative colitis.

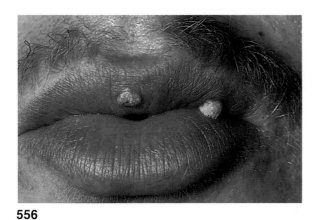

556

556 Verrucae vulgares

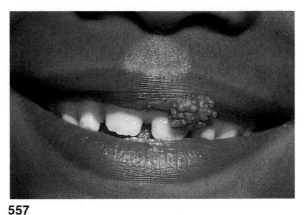

557

557 Papilloma of the upper lip
This is a typical mulberry form of a papilloma.

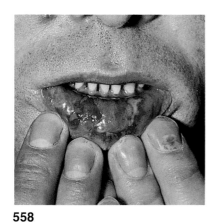

558

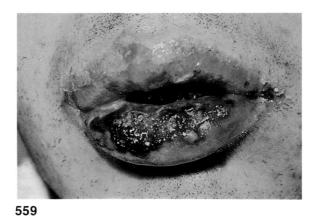

559

558–559 Erythema multiforme of the lip
The mucosa of the lower lip in this young adult shows an irregular erythematous lesion that extends slightly onto the buccal mucosa. The surface of the polycyclogyrate lesion is hemorrhagic laterally and fibroid medially, Fig.

558. – In Fig. **559** there is superficial ulceration and crusting on the lower lip. This lesion accompanied pulmonary pneumonia and was associated with balanitis, urethritis, and conjunctivitis.

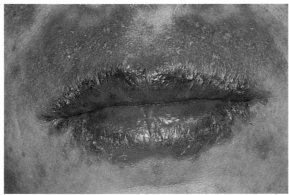

560

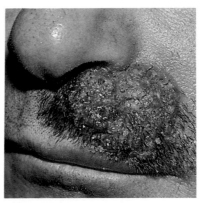

561

560 Lupus erythematosus of the lips

561 Trichophytosis of the upper lip
These pustular lesions are sharply circumscribed and covered with a crust of variable thickness. With tangential pressure, purulent exudate may be expressed from

the lesions. Hair shafts with edematous root sheaths can be extracted from each pustular lesion. A definitve etiologic diagnosis can be obtanined only by a culture demonstrating fungal elements (*Trichophyton tonsurans*).

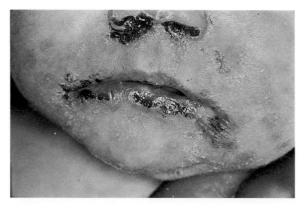

562

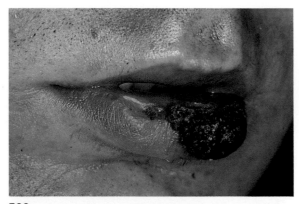

563

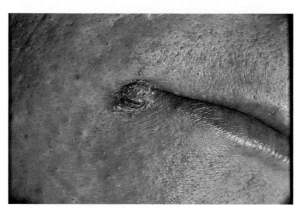

564

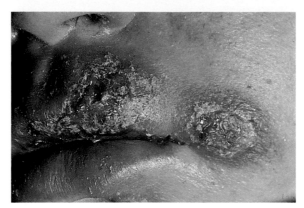

565

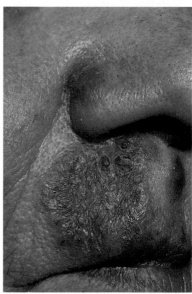

566

562–566 Syphilis

In this infant with congenital lues Fig. **562** there is a coryza associated with flat infiltrates in the nose and mouth. There is fissuring at the corner of the left side of the mouth. – Fig. **563** is a primary lesion of syphilis of the lower lip. Luetic primaries lead to a firm, indurated ulcer from which treponema pallidum can be easily isolated. Mucosal lesions occur in the mouth. – Fig. **564** demonstrates a crusted secondary luetic papule at the corner of the mouth. In this case of secondary lues there was generalized lymphadenopathy and a positive serologic reaction for syphilis. See Figs. **516** and **598** for other examples of secondary syphilis. – Fig. **565** demonstrates an impetigo-like form of secondary syphilis in a rapidly progressing form of the disease known as lues maligna. There are eroded, crusted ulcers in the upper lip and angle of the mouth. – Fig. **566** shows the tuberous stage of tertiary lues in the upper lip. Serologic tests were strongly positive.

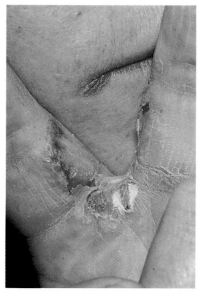

567

567 Intertriginous perlèche
Inflammatory lesions and fissure formation at the angle of the mouth with accumulations of whitish, macerated epithelium may be seen in malnourished children and edentulous adults or may be of mycotic origin. In this patient the condition was associated with lesions in the web of the fingers (erosio interdigitalis blastomycetica).

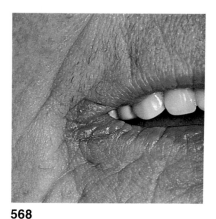

568

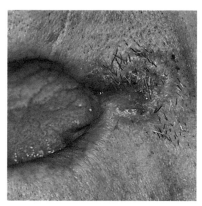

569

568 Acanthosis nigricans
There is a thickened perlèche of the angles of the mouth.

569 Carcinoma at the corner of the mouth
There is an ulcerated granular lesion with an elevated indurated margin at the corner of the mouth. First thought to be perlèche, squamous cell carcinoma was diagnosed from a biopsy of the tissue.

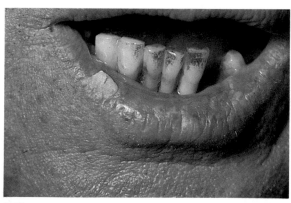

570

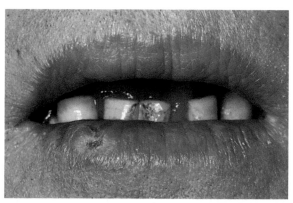

571

570 Leukoplakia of the lip
Such lesions usually occur at the site of chronic irritation and, as in this patient, are common in pipe smokers. A "white patch" of this type is not managed by clinical conjecture and its persistence merits excisional biopsy.

571 Early carcinoma of the lip
The lesion occupies the typical location between the outer and middle thirds of the lip and arises from atrophic epithelium, which proved upon excision to be squamous cell carcinoma.

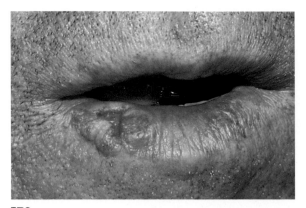

572

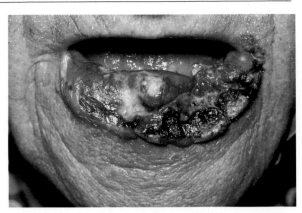

573

572–573 Squamous cell carcinomas of the lower lips, pipe-smoker's cancers

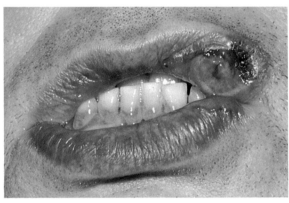

574

574 Squamous cell carcinoma of the upper lip
There is a moderately cornifying, poorly differentiated, squamous cell carcinoma of the left upper lip in this nonsmoker. There is a left submandibular lymph node metastasis. (Carcinomatous involvement of the upper lip is rare.)

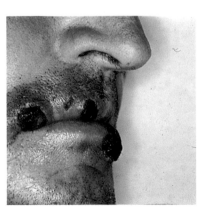

575

575 Acute leukemia
There are perioral and mucosal elevated, ulcerated, hemorrhagic and crusted leukemic infiltrates. The patient is 24 years old.

Diseases of the Floor of the Mouth

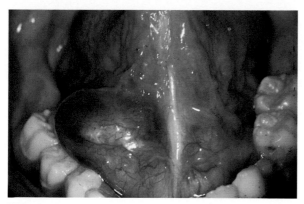

576

576 Ranula
Fig. **576** shows a ranula in the floor of the mouth of a seven-year-old child. There is a painless swelling under the tongue which interferes with speech. This cyst arises in the sublingual duct and contains mucous.

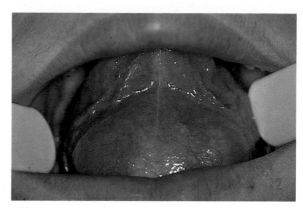

577

577 Sublingual dermoid cyst
This lesion is a teratoma in a 23-year-old patient.

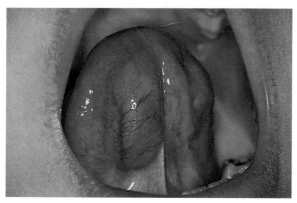

578

578 Nuhn-Blandin cyst
This lesion on the undersurface of the tip of the tongue is a retention cyst arising in the anterior lingual gland.

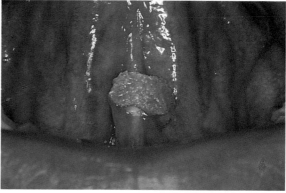

579

579 Mucosal papilloma of the frenulum
Histology of this lesion in a 21-year-old male was benign.

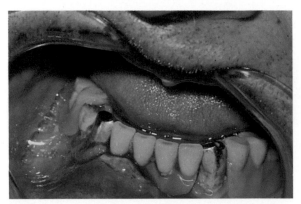

580

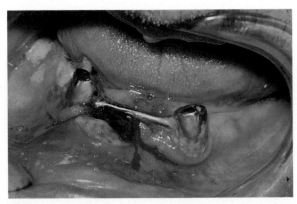

581

580–581 Squamous cell carcinoma of the alveolus
Fig. **580** shows a carcinoma on the alveolus in a denture wearer. Fig. **581** shows an exophytic, hemorrhagic car-

cinoma of the alveolus which lay under a dental bridge (same patient).

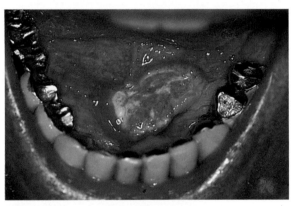

582

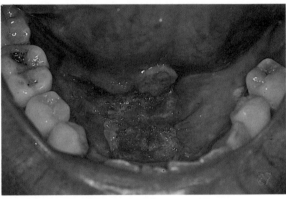

583

582–584 Squamous cell carcinomas of the floor of the mouth
There is extension to the undersurface of the tongue (Figs. **583, 584**). – The typical history of these patients: alcohol, tobacco and often badly neglected teeth.

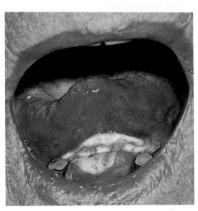

584

Diseases of the Tongue

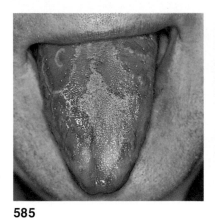

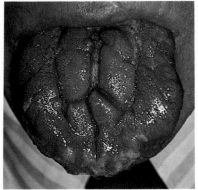

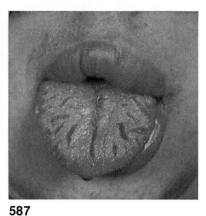

585

586

587

585 Geographic tongue

586–587 Lingua plicata
Fig. **586** shows a form of lingua plicata with macroglossia, lingua scrotalis, associated with the Melkersson-

Rosenthal syndrome. There is a secondary candida infection. In Fig. **587** the lingua plicata is also associated with the Melkersson-Rosenthal syndrome, but is less far advanced. There is an associated swelling of the lips and a left facial paralysis.

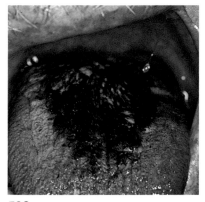

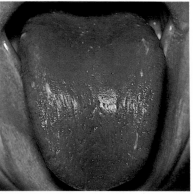

588

589

588 Black hairy tongue
Hyperkeratosis of the horny scales of the filiform lingual papillae occurs predominantly among adults, in the medial portion of the tongue, appearing as black or brown "fur." Causes of this condition are varied and may include local inflammatory processes in the mouth, use of irritating mouthwashes or lozenges, or alteration of vitamin B metabolism in the gastrointestinal tract resulting from antibiotic administration.

589 Glossitis (Möller-Hunter)
Smooth, irregular, somewhat depressed areas occur on the surface of the tongue. Distinct papillary markings of this type are most frequently associated with pernicious anemia; a similar glossitis can follow deficiency anemias, especially pellagra.

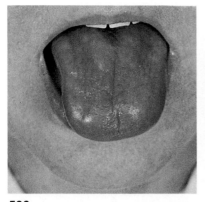

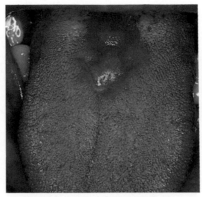

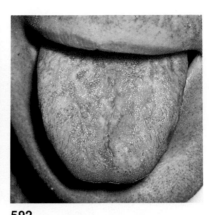

590   **591**   **592**

590 Glossitis with Sjögren syndrome

This 47-year-old female complained of dryness of the mouth and a burning sensation of the tongue. There was atrophy of the lingual and oral mucosa. The full-blown Sjögren's syndrome has, in addition, parotid swelling, keratoconjunctivitis, rheumatoid manifestations, and hypochronic anemia. The syndrome is confined chiefly to women.

591 Glossitis, rhomboid median type

Median rhomboid glossitis typically appears close to the foramen cecum and does not migrate, and is caused by persistance of the tuberculum impar.

592 Lichen planus of the tongue

Characteristic papular lesions may be observed on the mucosal surfaces of the tongue, mouth, and glans penis. The mucosal lesions are bluish or milky-white and occur in a striated or reticular pattern resembling cobwebs or fern leaves. Unlike Candida infections, the exudate cannot be easily wiped away.

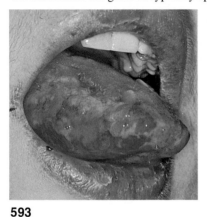

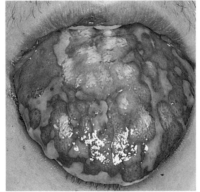

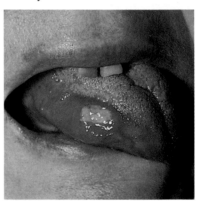

593   **594**   **595**

593 Pemphigus vulgaris of the tongue

There are serrated, defined, bright red erosions with gray-white remnants of ruptured blebs.

594 Erythema multiforme, exudativum

The etiology of this disorder is varied. There are idiopathic and symptomatic forms. Ingestion of certain medications or sensitization to bacterial antigens follow-ing a virus infection may cause the disease. In this patient the glossitis followed an herpetic virus infection.

595 Aphthous ulcer of the tongue

There is an oval, sharply demarcated ulcer with a gray-white fibrinous membrane on the lateral surface of the tongue. These lesions at times are extremely painful.

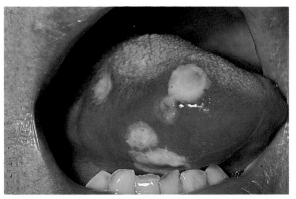

596

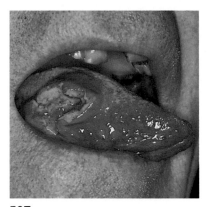

597

596 Lingual manifestations of Behçet's syndrome
Behçet's syndrome is a chronic illness characterized by chronic aphthous ulcerations of the mouth and genitalia, thrombophlebitis, erythema nodosum, neurologic symptoms and iritis with hypopyon. A chronic recurrent stomatitis as shown here may be the first symptom of this disorder.

597 Ulcerative tuberculosis of the tongue
The patient had active pulmonary tuberculosis, but a biopsy was necessary to rule out carcinoma.

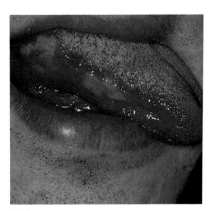

598

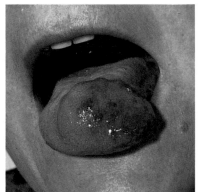

599

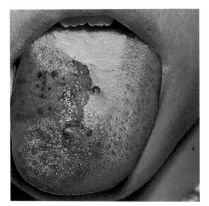

600

598 Secondary syphilis
There are opalescent luetic plaques on the lingual margin. Such lesions are highly infectious, see Figs **516, 562–566**.

599 Congenital hemangioma of the tongue
The patient is 45-years-old and has had this lesion of the tongue since birth.

600 Lymphangioma circumscripta
This 11-year-old patient had this lesion since birth. Biopsy showed a small cystic lymphangioma with fibroepithelial hyperplasia.

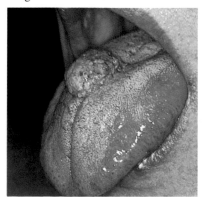

601

601 Papilloma of the tongue
The lesion of this 44-year-old patient was excised. Although clinically resembling carcinoma, the lesion was histologically reported to be papillary epithelium of the tongue with lymphocytic infiltration.

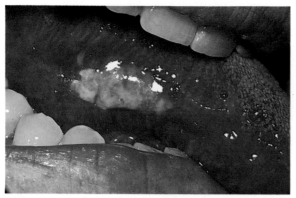

602

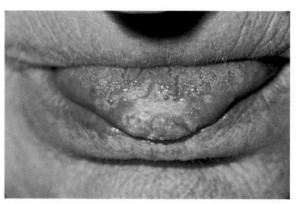

603

602 Leukoplakia
Lesions such as this one in a 48-year-old female may be precancerous and should be treated with excisional biopsy. No malignancy was noted histologically in this lesion although there was basal cell hyperplasia with indistinct margins.

603 Carcinoma in situ of the tip of the tongue
Excision biopsy of the lesion showed carcinoma in situ.

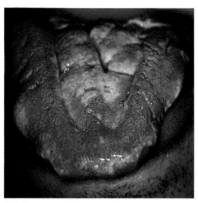

604

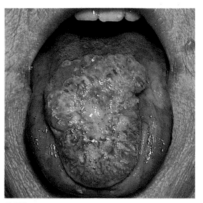

605

604 Leukoplakia of the mucosa of the tongue and oral mucosa
The severity of the leukoplakia with deformity and inflammation of the tongue predisposes to malignant degeneration. Biopsy was negative for malignancy. The patient smoked heavily.

605 Beginning malignant degeneration of tongue tumor
This 5 x 3 cm fungating tumor lies on the surface of the tongue of a 70-year-old female. The lesion enlarged slowly over a period of 6 years. There were no palpable cervical lymph nodes. There is leukoplakia of the tongue at the margin of the tumor. The lesion was removed by excisional biopsy. The histopathology report showed leukoplakia with deep epithelial papillae and atypical nuclei and dyskeratosis of single cells. There was a marked cellular reaction in the surrounding stroma. This is an example of beginning malignant degeneration.

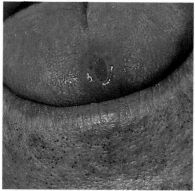

606

606 Squamous cell carcinoma of the tongue
There is a small carcinoma on the tip of the tongue of this 68-year-old male. A primary luetic lesion was ruled out by dark field studies and biopsy.

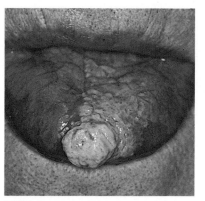

607

607 Carcinoma of the tip of the tongue
This lesion developed on the site of previous, long-standing leukoplakia. Biopsy showed it to be a squamous cell carcinoma. The patient smoked a pipe constantly.

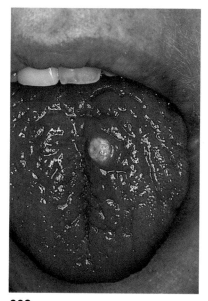

608

608 Squamous cell carcinoma
The carcinoma lies adjacent to the midline and arose in a lingua plicata.

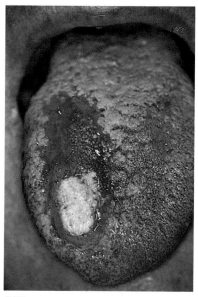

609

609 Squamous cell carcinoma
This 65-year-old male smoker noted a "white patch" on his tongue which he thought was due to a burn. Increasing pain and induration around the lesion brought him to the physician. Biopsy followed. Histology showed squamous cell carcinoma and leukoplakia.

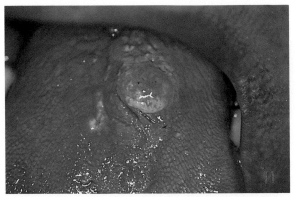

610

610 Squamous cell carcinoma of the tongue
This 40-year-old patient smoked and drank heavily.
There is an elevated carcinoma and leukoplakia on the
posterior surface of the tongue adjacent to the midline.
There were bilateral cervical metastases.

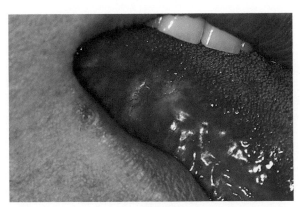

611

611 Squamous cell carcinoma of the tongue
The hard infiltrating lesion of the lateral aspect of the
tongue has a raised margin surrounding a central,
densely scarred indentation.

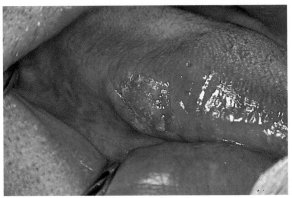

612

**612 Squamous cell carcinoma of the lateral margin of
　　the tongue**
There were submandibular metastases associated with
this carcinoma in a 56-year-old heavy smoker and
drinker.

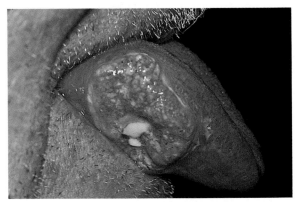

613

613 Exophytic squamous cell carcinoma
The patient, a 79-year-old hotelier, had bilateral fixed
cervical metastases.

Diseases of the Oral Mucosa and Gingiva

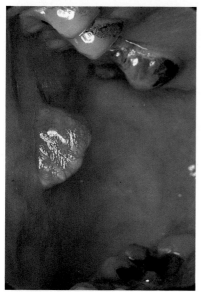

614

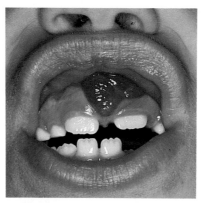

615

614 Proptosis of the buccal mucosa
Fibrous buccal mucosa has swollen to fill the gap caused by an extracted tooth.

615 Telangiectatic granuloma of the gingiva
The lesion arose in this 6-year-old child following an injury from a nail.

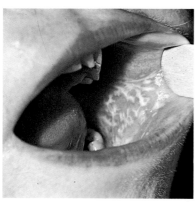

616

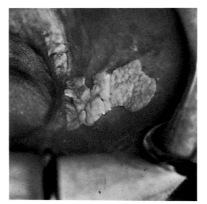

617

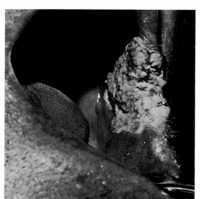

618

616 Lichen ruber planus of the oral mucosa
Bluish-white reticulated formations are present. In this nonerosive form, a network of fine or thick, violaceous, interlacing lines shows a variety of patterns. This condition may be associated with lesions of the flexor aspects of the skin of the wrists and forearms.

617 Leukoplakia of the buccal mucosa
This 54-year-old edentulous female patient was a heavy smoker. There is leukoplakia within the buccal mucosa, on the lower alveolar ridge, and on the anterior palatine arch. This lesion was asymptomatic.

618 Squamous cell carcinoma arising from leukoplakia
The lesion arises from precancerous leukoplakia on the mucosa of the corner of the mouth. The patient was a 57-year-old pipe-smoker.

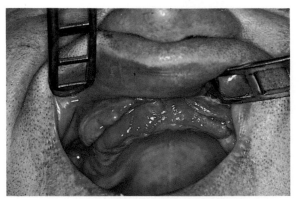

619

619 Papillary hyperplasia of the upper alveolar ridge
Intense overgrowth (hyperplasia) of the upper gum was produced by an ill-fitting denture. The lesion was benign on biopsy.

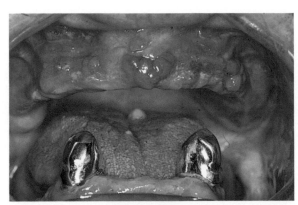

620

620 Morbus Pringle with hyperplastic gingivitis
The patient has taken antiepileptic medication for many years.

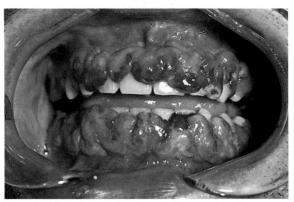

621

621 Gingival hyperplasia with myeloblastic leukemia
Gingival hypertrophy, such as shown here, often is the first clinical manifestation of a blood dyscrasia. This patient had myeloblastic leukemia.

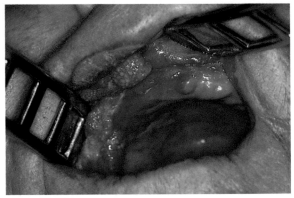

622

622 Squamous cell carcinoma of the gingiva
Exuberant, nodular, easily bleeding tumor masses occupy the gingival and adjacent buccal mucosa. There was osteolysis of the alveolar bone.

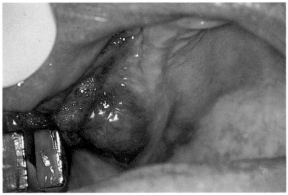

623

623 Squamous cell carcinoma of the upper alveolar ridge, right
There is spread into the maxillary sinus. The patient stated that her dentures did not fit properly for the past five months.

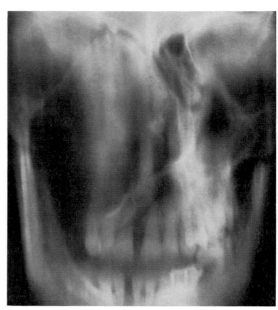

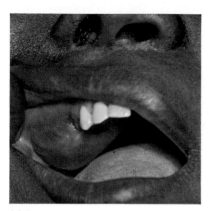

624

625

624–625 Adamantinoma
Fig. **624** shows a smooth mass projecting from the alveolar process and roof of the mouth which proved, on biopsy, to be an adamantinoma or ameloblastoma. These tumors usually arise in the mandible and are rarely malignant. Lesions of the maxilla can lead to fistulas of the maxillary sinus. Clinical differentiation must be made from carcinoma, osteitis fibrosa, and luetic gumma. – Fig. **625** is a tomograph of this patient which shows erosion of the tumor into the orbit with destruction of the walls of the maxillary sinus and extension into the right nasal cavity.

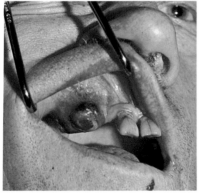

626 Malignant melanoma of the upper alveolar ridge, right
There was destruction of the bone of the neighboring portions of the maxillary sinus, as shown radiographically.

626

Diseases of the Palate

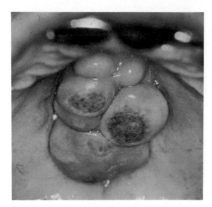

627

627 Torus palatinus
There is superfical mucosal ulceration.

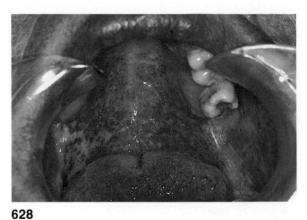

628

628 Drug reaction of the palate and buccal mucosa

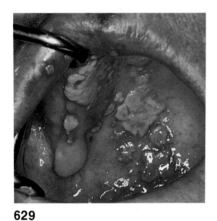

629

629 Herpes zoster of the palatal mucosa, right
The palatal lesions accompanied herpes zoster oticus of the same side. See Figs **34–36**.

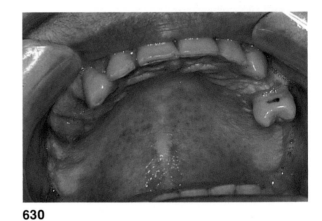

630

630 Leukokeratosis nicotinica of the palate
The hard palate is involved in a somewhat verrucous, gray-white discoloration which extends to the alveolar crests. The ducts of the minor salivary glands are reddened. The patient was a chain smoker.

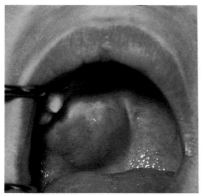

631

631 Mixed tumor, pleomorphic adenoma of the palate, right
There is a firm, non-inflamed mass arising from the soft palate.

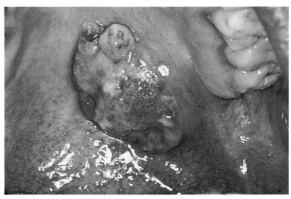

632

632 Adenocystic carcinoma of the palate, left
This superficially ulcerated lesion arose from the minor salivary glands of the hard palate in a 37-year-old male.

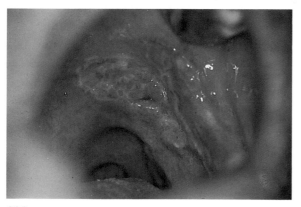

633

633 Squamous cell carcinoma of the soft palate, left
This 55-year-old patient "smoked like a chimney" and "drank like a fish."

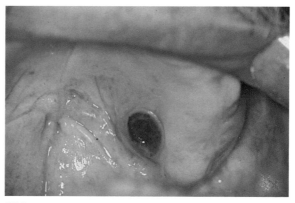

634

634 Squamous cell carcinoma of the hard palate, left
This lesion arose from chronic irritation caused by a poorly fitting denture. The first clinical diagnosis was pressure ulcer, but biopsy showed carcinoma.

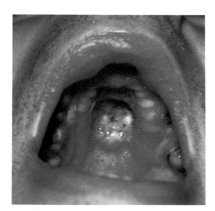

635

635 Midline lethal granuloma
This 46-year-old male had presented himself a year before with purulent rhinitis. Examination revealed complete destruction of the nasal septum as well as a 2 cm necrotizing lesion of the hard palate. This disorder, when associated with specific pulmonary and renal lesions, constitutes the components of Wegener's granulomatosis. See Figs **322–324**.

Diseases
of the Larynx

Clinical Anatomy

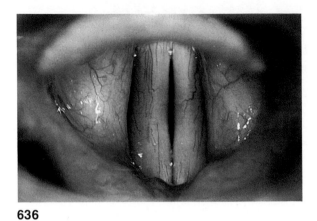

636

636 Magnifying mirror laryngoscopy
The normal larynx in phonation.

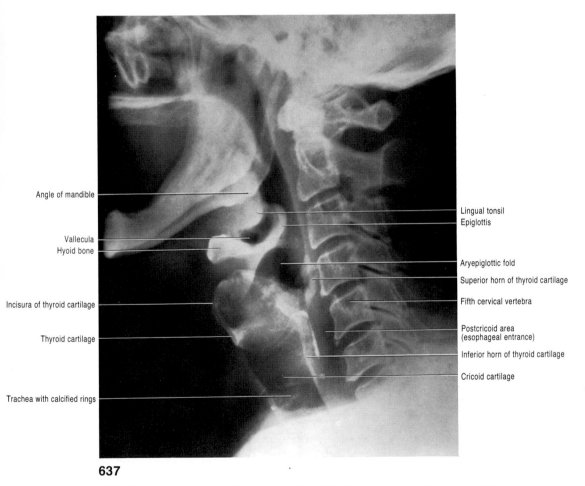

Angle of mandible

Vallecula
Hyoid bone

Incisura of thyroid cartilage

Thyroid cartilage

Trachea with calcified rings

Lingual tonsil
Epiglottis

Aryepiglottic fold

Superior horn of thyroid cartilage

Fifth cervical vertebra

Postcricoid area
(esophageal entrance)

Inferior horn of thyroid cartilage

Cricoid cartilage

637

637 The normal laryngeal structures identified in a lateral radiogram of the neck

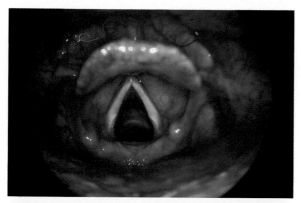

638

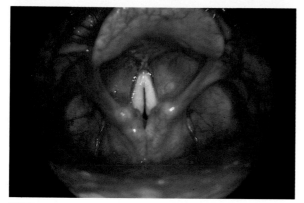

639

638–639 90°-telescopic views of the larynx during in-
spiration and phonation
During inspiration, Fig. **638**, the vallecula, vocal cords,
and subglottic space are clearly seen. With phonation,
Fig. **639**, the piriform sinuses and the postcricoid region
become visible.

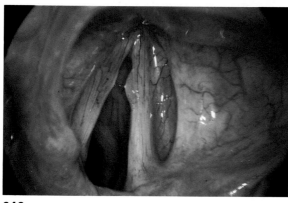

640

640 Laryngeal ventricle, right
The ventricle is clearly seen. There is a vocal nodule on
the phonating edge of the true cord with a slight reaction
on the opposite cord.

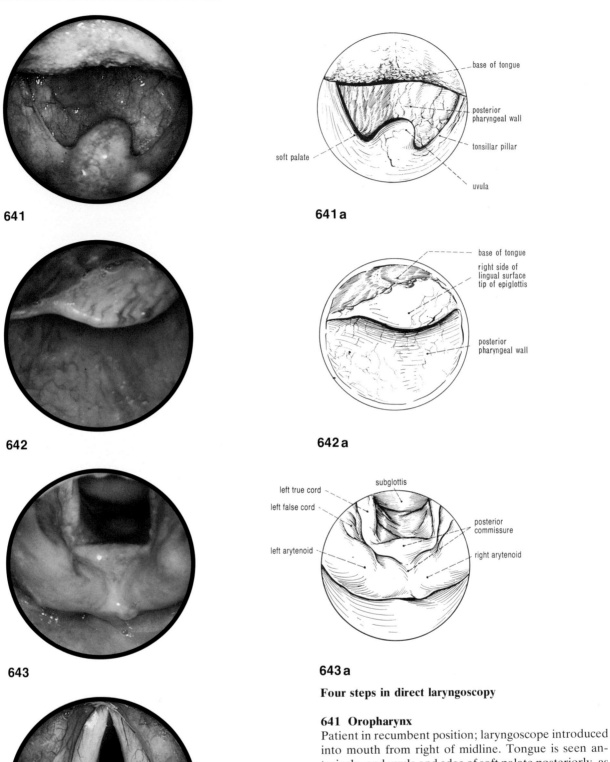

641

641a

base of tongue

posterior
pharyngeal wall

tonsillar pillar

soft palate

uvula

642

642a

base of tongue

right side of
lingual surface

tip of epiglottis

posterior
pharyngeal wall

643

643a

left true cord

subglottis

left false cord

posterior
commissure

left arytenoid

right arytenoid

644

Four steps in direct laryngoscopy

641 Oropharynx
Patient in recumbent position; laryngoscope introduced
into mouth from right of midline. Tongue is seen anteriorly, and uvula and edge of soft palate posteriorly, as
laryngoscope exposes midportion of posterior wall of
oropharynx.

642 Tip of epiglottis
Laryngoscope advanced along tongue to expose right
side of tip of epiglottis.

643 Posterior commissure
Blade of laryngoscope dips under edge of epiglottis, is
advanced approximately 1 cm, and then lifted anteriorly
to expose posterior commissure.

644 Glottis (inspiration)
With patient's occiput lifted anteriorly, glottis is visualized so as to show edges of true and false cords, anterior and posterior commissures, and interior of upper
portion of trachea.

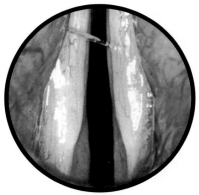

645

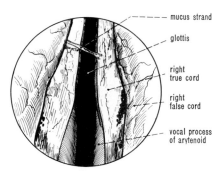

645 a

645 The glottis following phonation
The parallel cords, relaxed after phonation of "E", lie close to the midline. A strand of mucous extends from one cord to the other anteriorly. Pink mucosa covers the vocal processes of the arytenoid posteriorly.

Congenital Anomalies

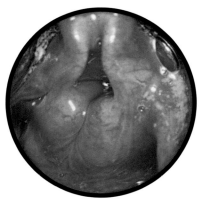

646

646 a

646 Laryngomalacia in a newborn
There is a spasmodic closure of the larynx in the inspiratory phase of respiration. The curled, soft epiglottis and the arytenoids are drawn into and obstract the glottis.

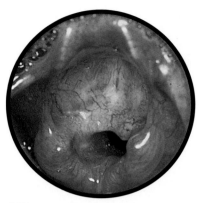

647

647 Congenital supraglottic laryngeal web
The larynx of a one-day-old infant. The cry was absent, dyspnea and stridor were marked. The false cords are sealed in the midline except for a small airway posteriorly. During phonation inward movement of the arytenoids closed the airway completely.

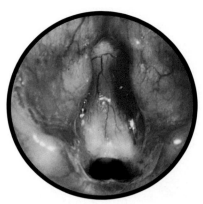

648

648 Congenital membranous glottic web
8-year-old boy with husky, almost inaudible voice. Tracheostomy for extreme dyspnea had been done in infancy. There is only a small aperture in the posterior glottis.

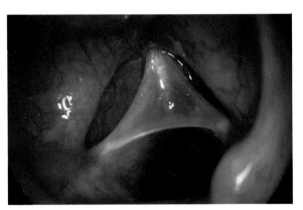

649

649 Congenital glottic web
The patient is a 21-year-old female who had a falsetto voice since infancy.

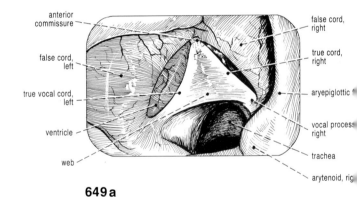

649a

anterior commissure

false cord, left

true vocal cord, left

ventricle

web

false cord, right

true cord, right

aryepiglottic f

vocal process right

trachea

arytenoid, rig

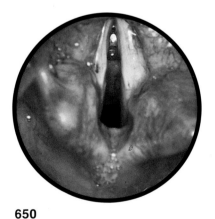

650

650 Congenital subglottic stenosis
Subglottic stenosis in infant 3 months of age, consisting of a cricoid cartilage deformity involving the anterior half of the cartilage.

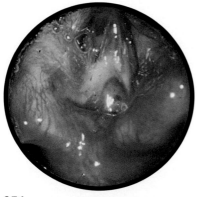

651

651 Congenital laryngeal atresia
Infant, one year of age. An emergency tracheotomy was done at birth because, in spite of extreme efforts at respiration, the infant was obstructed and emitted no cry. The outlines of the cords appear through the transparent membranous web.

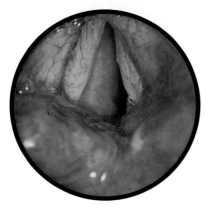

652

652a

652 Congenital subglottic stenosis
Subglottic stenosis of the larynx of a 9-month-old infant with stridor since birth. A tracheotomy had been performed during an acute episode of laryngotracheobron-

chitis and extubation was delayed because of the persistence of this subglottic swelling left. The cords themselves moved poorly, cushioned by the approximation of the subglottic tissues (congenital haemangioma).

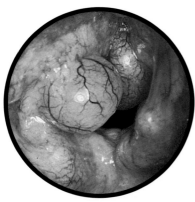

653

653a

653 Congenital cysts of the larynx
The larynx of a one-week-old infant. Extreme stridor and dyspnea, and a high-pitched, squeaky cry were indications for the laryngoscopy. The motility of the cords was decreased by the bulk of the cysts, which prevented their approximation.

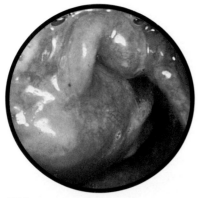

654

654–655 Congenital laryngocele

A newborn infant with stridor and dyspnea, and without a cry. A large cystic mass is seen occupying the left side of the larynx. The left aryepiglottic fold, false cord, and arytenoid are covered as the cyst fills the left piriform sinus and the glottis itself. The epiglottis is edematous and partially compressed by the cyst. A tracheostomy was done in the first hour after birth. – A lateral radiogram of the neck shows a large cystic mass in the region of the larynx Fig. **655**. The tip of the epiglottis and the laryngeal ventricle itself can be identified. The trachea is within normal limits.

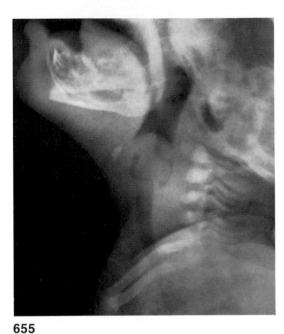

655

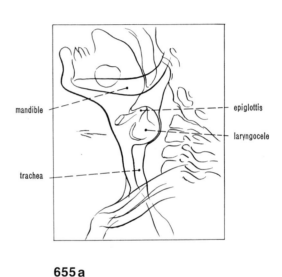

655 a

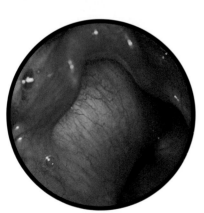

656

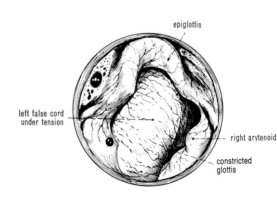

656 a

656 Congenital laryngocele, inspiration

Extremely dyspneic cyanotic infant, one week of age, whose cry was only an occasional squeak. Laryngoscopy shows a congenital cyst protruding from the left laryngeal ventricle, classified as an internal laryngocele.

The left false cord is drawn extremely taut as the cyst bulges under it, covering the right false and true cords. On deep inspiration a small airway is apparent just anterior to the right arytenoid.

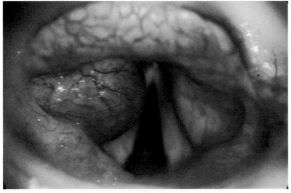

657

657 Unilateral internal laryngocele
A 62-year-old woman developed hoarseness and intermittent dyspnea. The mirror view of the larynx shows cystic enlargement of the right false cord. When the patient coughed or talked forcefully, the mass increased in size to overhang the right true cord. On direct laryngoscopy the mass was found to contain thick viscid fluid. Dyspnea followed each cough as the laryngocele inflated; the glottic lumen returned to normal size as it gradually deflated.

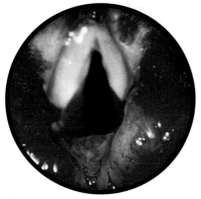

658

658 Congenital hemangioma of the larynx
Laryngeal involvement of an extensive "port wine" congenital hemangioma of the face, scalp, and oral cavity in an infant 6 months of age.

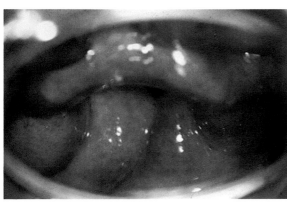

659

660

659 Angioneurotic edema of the larynx
A woman, 24 years of age, had had recurring attacks of sudden swelling of various portions of lips and cheeks (see Fig. 319). More recently she had developed severe hoarseness rapidly progressing to aphonia and dyspnea. Edema of the epiglottis, aryepiglottic folds, and particularly of the arytenoids prevents visualization of the cords (mirror view).

660 Bilateral recurrent laryngeal nerve paralysis post-arytenoidectomy
A 46-year-old woman who had had two thyroidectomies "lost" her voice following the first operation and became severely dyspneic after the second. A right intralaryngeal arytenoidectomy was performed, reestablishing an adequate airway. The right cord is seen in a semiabducted position (mirror view).

Laryngeal Trauma

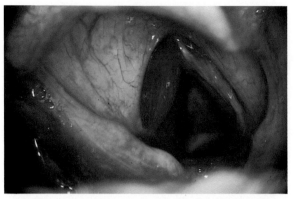

661

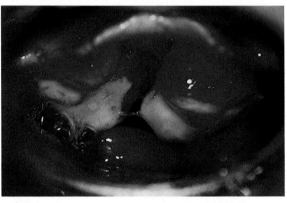

662

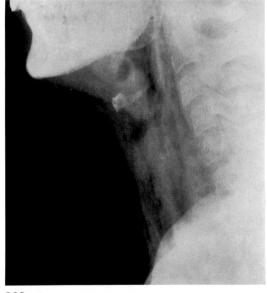

663

661 Blunt laryngeal trauma
There is a hematoma of the left vocal cord, the right sub-glottic area, and the left side of the pharynx, 90°-telescopic view.

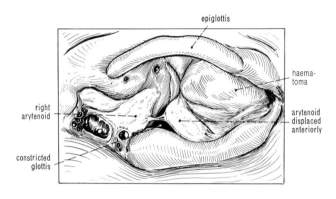

662a

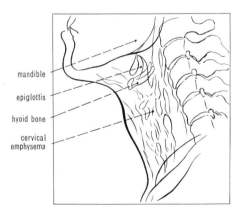

663a

662–663 Fracture of the larynx
The patient was a 31-year-old woman seen one week after injury in an automobile accident. She was the front seat passenger and her head had struck the windshield and her neck, the edge of the dashboard. All structures are seen to be edematous and hemorrhagic, and there was extensive subcutaneous crepitant emphysema. The arytenoids are dislocated and displaced forward under the epiglottis, compressing the aryepiglottic folds. The airway is seriously impaired. An emergency tracheotomy was performed following the accident. Subcutaneous as well as retropharyngeal emphysema is evident in the radiogram (Fig. **663**), obliterating the normal laryngeal and tracheal contour.

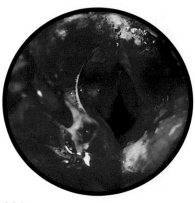

664

664 Acute laryngeal hematoma
This 21-year-old man was the victim of an attempted strangling. Hemorrhage into the soft tissues of the entire larynx was most severe in the left aryepiglottic fold and arytenoid. Edema and hemorrhage into the cords diminish the airway.

Laryngeal Trauma from Intubation

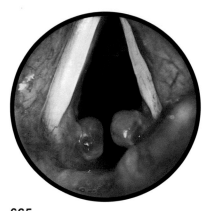

665

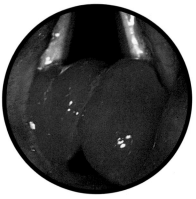

666

665–666 Granulomas of the vocal cords following endotracheal anesthesia
This 40-year-old patient suffered hoarseness, cough and discomfort in her throat six weeks following endotracheal anesthesia. The discrete granulomas lie in the typical position over the ulcerated surfaces of the vocal processes of both arytenoids.

This 33-year-old female noted increasing hoarseness dating from an endotracheal anesthesia two months before. The two large granulomas, arising from the vocal processes of the arytenoids, move in and out with respiration and prevent approximation of the vocal cords.

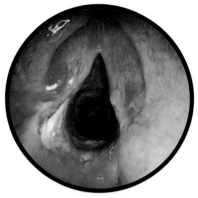

667

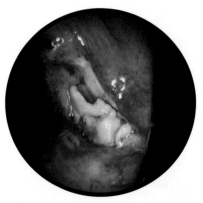

668

667 Laryngeal trauma following endotracheal intubation

Due to drug overdosage, this 40-year-old male was intubated for 10 days. Following extubation there is a synechia at the anterior commissure involving the anterior one-fourth of each vocal cord. The vocal cords are edematous, and there is pressure necrosis of the mucosa overlying each vocal process.

668 Necrosis and fracture arytenoid cartilage, right

The mucosa overlying the arytenoid has sloughed away exposing this fracture and necrosis of the cartilage which followed an endotracheal intubation of seven days duration. The glottis lies at the left of the photograph.

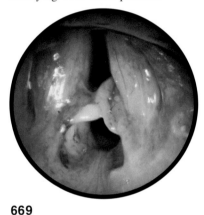

669

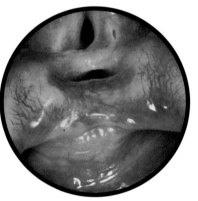

670

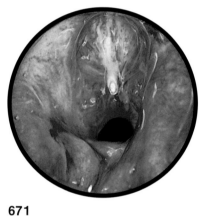

671

669 Intubation granuloma and early synechia

This 18-year-old patient suffered multiple traumatic lesions in an auto accident. Following a six day intubation the vocal cords are edematous and thickened. There are granulomas at each vocal process and a beginning synechia of the cords where the granulomas appose each other.

670 Interarytenoid synechia

Following prolonged intubation this five month old infant developed this fibrous synechia between the arytenoid processes which fixed the vocal cords. The entrance of the esophagus is visible inferiorly.

671 Synechia of the vocal cords

This fibrous scar stenosing the glottis occurred in a seven-year-old boy following prolonged endotracheal intubation of one month.

Vocal Trauma

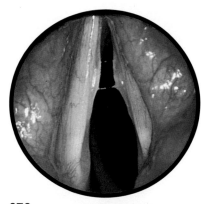

672

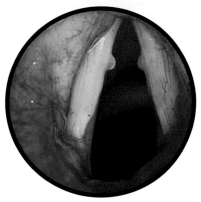

673

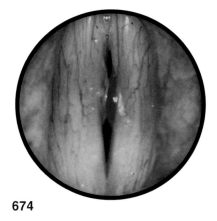

674

672 Vocal nodules, "singer's nodes"
This 28-year-old mother of five children had been intermittently hoarse for three years. She had a loud, demanding voice, apparently abusing it in her efforts to discipline the children. The soft sessile nodules appear as **edematous** swellings, most prominently at the junction of the anterior and middle third of each cord. Thin strands of mucus bridge the glottis between the nodules.

673 Vocal nodules, "singer's nodes"
These **fibrous** nodules lie on the typical location on the vocal cords.

674 Vocal nodules
The vocal cords are thickened, the vascular pattern is prominent, and the nodules themselves are discrete, soft, and hemorrhagic. The manner in which they create an air loss on phonation is evident.

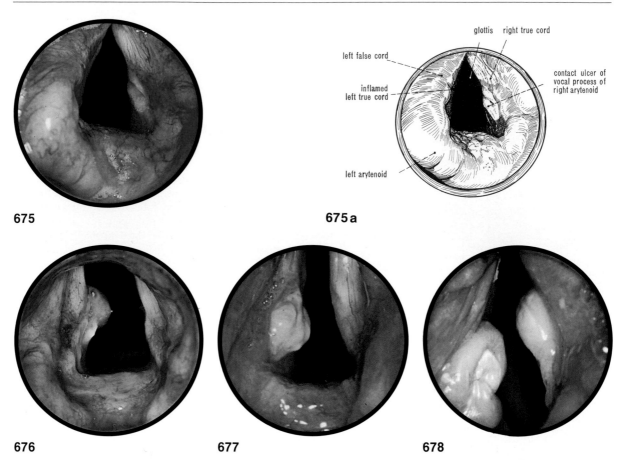

675

675a

glottis right true cord

left false cord

inflamed
left true cord

contact ulcer of
vocal process of
right arytenoid

left arytenoid

676   **677**   **678**

675–678 Contact ulcers of the larynx

Contact ulcers are uni-or bilateral, superficial ulcerative lesions of the mucosa, overlying the vocal processes of the arytenoids, the pars intercartilaginea of the glottis. They occur most often in males and are caused by vocal abuse. Continued misuse of the larynx may lead to granulomas and hyperplasia at the site of the lesions. Acute ulcer of the right vocal process: the patient, a 44-year-old preacher in a large congregation, complained of pain and tenderness in the right side of the neck at the level of the lateral border of the thyroid cartilage. Pain, accentuated on swallowing, radiated to the right ear, increasing as the day progressed. Noteworthy are the inflammatory zone around the border of the ulcer and vascularity of the opposite cord, Fig. **675**. – A 37-year-old political candidate was engaged in a heated campaign. He developed hoarseness and pain, especially on swal-

lowing, in the left side of the neck at the level of the posterior inferior border of the thyroid cartilage, radiating to the left ear. The tip of the left vocal process shows a small area of necrosis in addition to the granuloma. Vascularity of both arytenoids is increased, Fig. **676**. – An exudate-covered granuloma of a contact ulcer of the left arytenoid was observed in a 39-year-old salesman. Constant telephoning, much of it long distance, with use of a harsh, rapid, rasping type of speech characterized his selling technique, Fig. **677**. – Large contact ulcer granulomas in a 46-year-old salesman who talked constantly in noisy surroundings. Hoarseness and pain in the throat on talking and swallowing progressed as the day went on. The large, soft granulomas are seen to approximate on phonation, fitting into each other to surround the exudate-covered base of the ulcers, which are centered over the tips of the vocal processes, Fig. **678**.

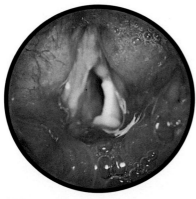

679

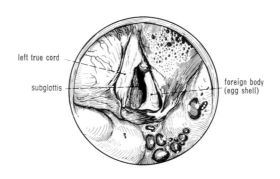

left true cord

subglottis

foreign body (egg shell)

679a

679 Foreign body in the larynx
A piece of eggshell was discovered in the larynx of a 10-month-old infant who had suddenly choked while

being fed a soft-boiled egg. Stridor and dyspnea increased during the following days with voice changes progressing to aphonia.

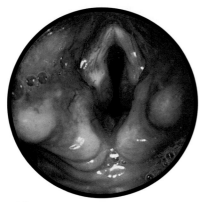

680

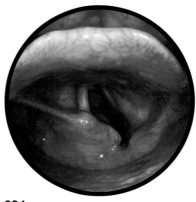

681

680 Bilateral central superior and recurrent laryngeal paralysis
The child has a meningoencephalocele and hydrocephalus. Paralysis of the superior laryngeal nerves prevents tensing of the vocal cords by the cricothyroid muscle. The cords are flaccid and the voice breathy and weak.

681 Recurrent laryngeal nerve paralysis, left
The arytenoid cartilage is displaced anteriorly and the left vocal cord fixed in a paramedian position.

Inflammatory Diseases

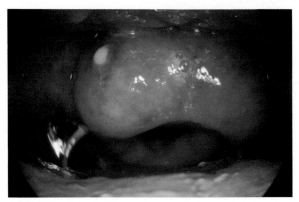

682

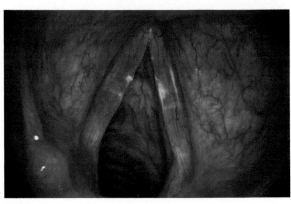

683

682 Abscess of the epiglottis
The abscess is about to rupture spontaneously. – Acute epiglottitis, especially in children, can cause rapid onset of dyspnea which can cause suffocation.

683 Acute laryngitis
There is marked injection of the entire endolarynx. The vocal cords are slightly edematous, inflamed and, a thin layer of mucous covers both cords.

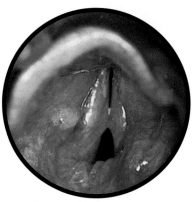

684

684 Acute laryngitis
In this case the chronic inflammatory process, leading to edema and thickening, involves the false and true cords, extending to the posterior surface of the epiglottis as well as to the posterior commissure of the larynx.

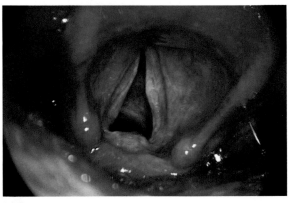

685

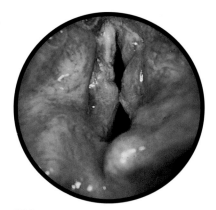

686

685 Chronic laryngitis
This 57-year-old male was a heavy smoker who was exposed to industrial fumes. Hoarseness for several years. The vocal cords are injected and edematous, and the mucosa of the middle thirds, especially on the right side, is thickened.

686 Chronic hypertrophic laryngitis
Markedly thickened, irregular cord edges in a 42-year-old man. The patient smoked excessively, kept his home exceedingly hot and dry, and constantly abused his voice by forced loud talking. Histology: Extensive dysplasia and many atypical nuclei in the epithelial cells.

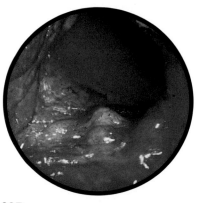

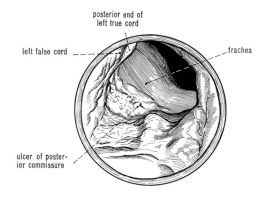

posterior end of
left true cord

left false cord

trachea

ulcer of poster-
ior commissure

687

687a

687 Chronic ulcerative laryngitis
This patient, a chemist, was exposed to acid fumes for varying periods of time and failed to take the usual re-

commended precautions. Hoarseness became severe and was associated with pain, dysphagia, and a sensation of dryness in the throat.

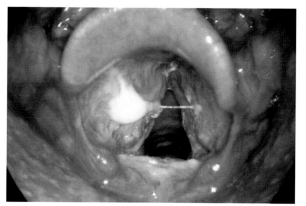

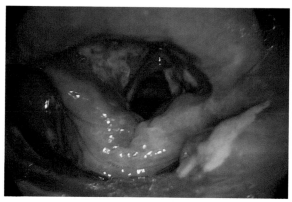

688

689

688 Chronic laryngitis sicca
There is diffuse hyperplasia of the mucosa in the glottic and subglottic areas, which are covered by crusted, dried mucous. The nose and nasopharynx were similarly involved and contributed to the pathology.

689 Postsurgical, postirradiation laryngitis
Following a frontolateral, partial resection, this 67-year-old patient received 6000 rads of radiotherapy. There is injection, swelling, and a membranous reaction of the arytenoid, and the postcricoid area. The endolarynx and the right lateral pharyngeal wall show fibrinous exudate. There was pain and dysphagia.

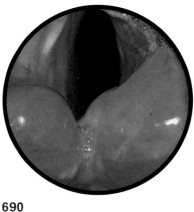

690 Postirradiation laryngeal edema
Edema of larynx in a 41-year-old woman followed treatment of a carcinoma of the left vocal cord. Hoarseness increased, with pain in the throat accentuated on swallowing; episodes of dyspnea and a sensation of dryness of the throat resulted. The arytenoids have a translucent swollen appearance, and the subglottic edema extended into the anterior commissure. The motility of the cords was impaired.

690

Specific Inflammatory Diseases

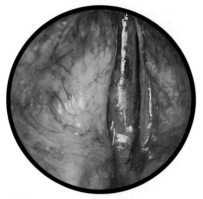

691

691 Unilateral tuberculous laryngitis

This 37-year-old man developed hoarseness gradually but progressively over a period of several months. The motility of both cords is normal, but the left cord is hyperemic and considerably thicker than the right. A chest radiogram revealed minimal tuberculosis of the right apex and the sputum contained acid-fast organisms. *Biopsy was necessary to rule out carcinoma.*

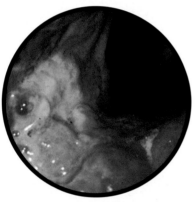

692

692 Tuberculous ulcer of the larynx

This 26-year-old man, who had far-advanced pulmonary tuberculosis, complained of pain radiating to the left ear, hoarseness, and dysphagia. Biopsy of the soft, exudate-covered ulcer as well as examination of the sputum confirmed the diagnosis.

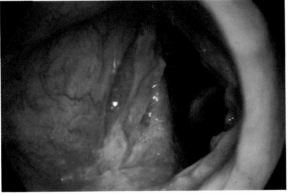

693

693 Tuberculosis of the larynx

There is a hyperplastic, ulcerated membranous lesion of the left vocal cord. The posterior portion of the right cord is also involved. Smear from the lesion revealed acid-fast bacilli.

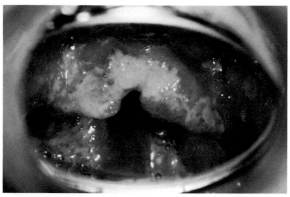

694

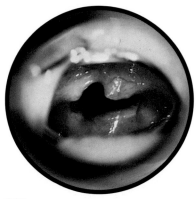

695

694–695 Ulcerative laryngeal tuberculosis
This 24-year-old patient had severe pain radiating to both ears, and dysphagia. Extensive ulceration was observed involving the epiglottis, aryepiglottic folds, and arytenoids. The destructive process caused the epiglottis to curl over the glottis itself and has denuded a portion of

the cartilaginous tip. The chest radiogram showed far advanced bilateral caseous tuberculosis, and the sputum contained tubercle bacilli. – Fig. **695** shows the larynx following treatment. The mucosa is smooth and the healed defect of the epiglottis is apparent.

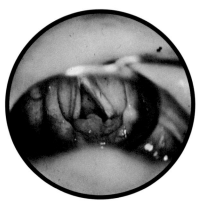

696

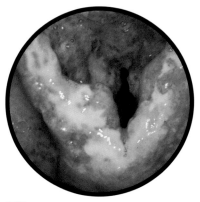

697

696 Tuberculoma of the larynx
The complaints of this 40-year-old man were hoarseness and pain in the throat of several weeks' duration. A chest radiogram showed an infiltrate in the right upper lobe with cavitation throughout the left lung. The mass in the posterior commissure and the sputum contained *M. tuberculosis*. (Figs. **694–696** mirror views.)

697 Tuberculosis of the larynx miliary
Miliary tuberculosis lesions involve the entire laryngeal and postcricoidal mucosa. The patient had far advanced pulmonary tuberculosis with phthisis.

Uncommon Diseases

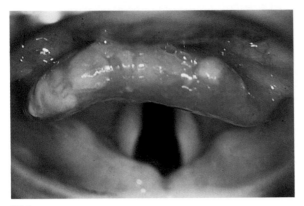

698

698 Pemphigus of the epiglottis
A woman, 34 years of age, complained of intermittent severe sore throats; painful vesicles appeared in the pharynx, ultimately rupturing and leaving an exudate-covered base. The lesions are seen to involve the tip of the epiglottis (s. Figs. **554** and **593**).

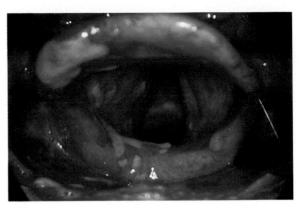

699

699 Herpes of the larynx
The patient was a 22-year-old student who complained of severe pain on swallowing and otalgia. Beside laryngeal lesions, similiar herpetic involvement occurs in the mouth and auricle. See Figs **629, 34, 35,** and **36.**

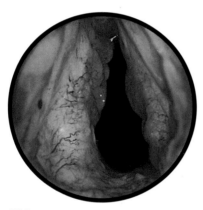

700

700 Amyloid disease of the larynx
Extensive amyloid tissue deposits on the left side of the larynx with a similar but less marked process under the

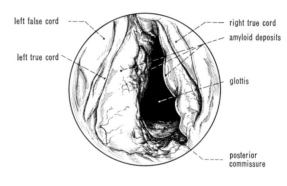

700 a

right cord. The patient, a 22-year-old man, had no other evidence of amyloid disease. Further investigation disclosed tracheopathia osteoplastica.

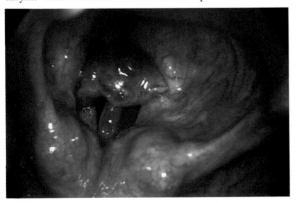

701

701 Amyloid tumor arising from the left vocal cord

Polyps

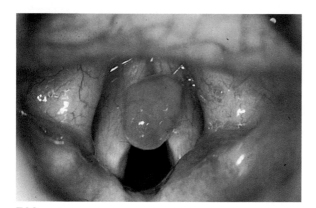

702

702 Polyp of the vocal cord, left

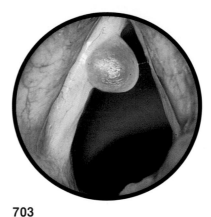

703

703 Polyp of the vocal cord
A polyp is attached along the phonating edge of the left vocal cord.

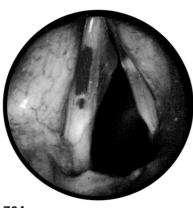

704

704 Hemorrhagic polyp vocal cord, left
Following severe vocal trauma and a rather sudden loss of voice, examination showed a hemorrhagic sessile polyp at the phonating edge of the left vocal cord. There are additional hemorrhages on the superior surface of the left and in the anterior third of the right vocal cords.

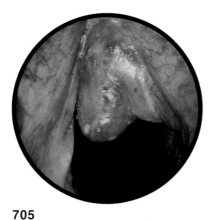

705

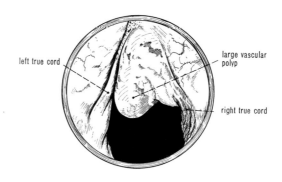

705a

705 Vascular polyp of the vocal cord
A large, vascular, sessile polyp occupies the anterior two-thirds of the right vocal cord. The patient was an ex-

tremely obese 54-year-old man with florid complexion and a deep guttural voice.

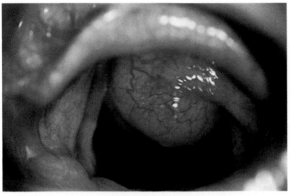

706

706 Polyp of the larynx
A huge pedunculated polyp is seen to arise from the left side of the larynx. The false as well as the true cord contribute to the origin of this polyp. The patient was a traffic policeman (mirror view).

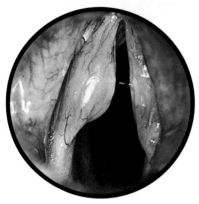

707

707 Sessile polyp of the vocal cord (beginning Reinke edema)
Persistent hoarseness of two years' duration was the complaint of a 42-year-old woman. Laryngoscopy demonstrated an edematous translucent polyp involving the anterior two-thirds of the left vocal cord. The right cord is similarly affected but additionally is superficially ulcerated along its phonating margin, the result of pressure by the left cord polyp during phonation.

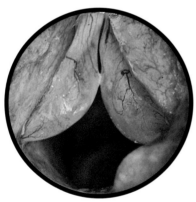

708

708 Chronic bilateral polypoid hypertrophic laryngitis; bilateral Reinke edema
The voice of this 52-year-old woman had been deep and rasping in quality and masculine in character. Stridor and dyspnea were noted after prolonged voice use. She was a heavy smoker.

Papilloma

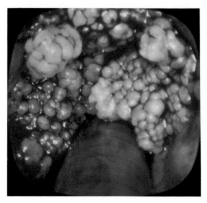

709

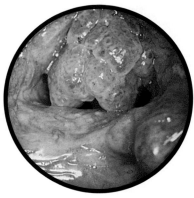

710

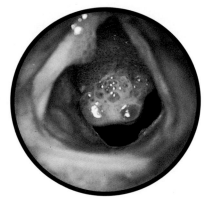

711

709 Papillomatosis of the larynx
Multiple papillomas are spread throughout the larynx, obstructing the lumen. The endotracheal tube is in the lower portion of the photograph.

710 Papilloma of the larynx
A large mass of papilloma is observed in the larynx of this 2-year-old child. He was extremely dyspneic and the

papilloma moved in and out of the glottis with each phase of the respiratory cycle.

711 Papilloma of the larynx and trachea
Pedunculated papillomas attached to the anterior tracheal wall, originating at the level of the first tracheal ring. A small solitary papilloma is observed to arise from the phonating edge of the left vocal cord.

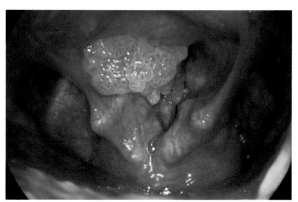

712

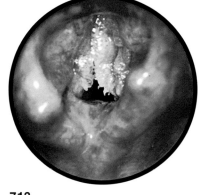

713

712 Papillomatosis of the larynx
The supraglottic area is covered with papillomas in this adult larynx. Histology was negative for carcinoma.

713 Hyperkeratotic papillomatosis of the larynx
16-month-old infant.

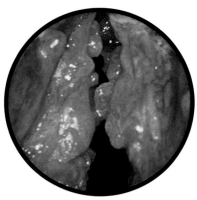

714

714 Multiple papillomas of the larynx
The larynx of a 42-year-old woman who had been hoarse all her adult life and had had laryngeal papillomas removed repeatedly over a period of 20 years. During each of five pregnancies, the papillomas disappeared.

Benign Tumors

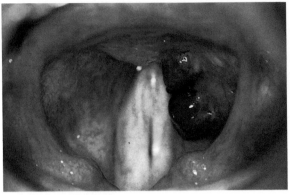

715

715 Hemangiomas of the left false cord
An incidental finding in a man 65 years of age who had no laryngeal symptoms. There are two rather large hemangiomas involving the left false cord. No other similar findings in the pharynx or larynx were noted. The rim of the laryngeal mirror is visible at the margins of the photograph.

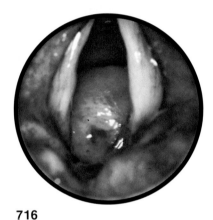

716

716 Subglottic fibroma
A 56-year-old woman who was dyspneic complained of an audible asthmatoid wheeze. A round pedunculated tumor, a fibroma, was seen that almost completely filled the airway. It was attached posteriorly to the anterior wall of the cricoid plate and disappeared from mirror view on inspiration. During phonation or with coughing, it rose to the cord level, causing a ball valve-like obstruction of the airway.

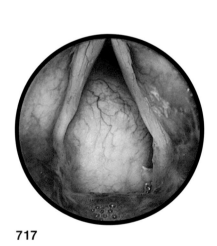

717

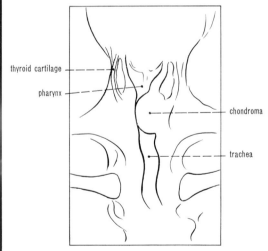

718

717–718 Subglottic chondroma of the larynx
Extreme dyspnea necessitated a tracheotomy in this 78-year-old woman: The tumor was smooth, quite symmetrical, and firm, and cord motility was only moderately impaired. A lateral radiogram of the larynx demonstrated a dense, smooth, round subglottic mass. The anteroposterior laminogram shows the mass to be attached to the left side of the cricoid cartilage (Fig. **718**).

Malignant and Premalignant Tumors

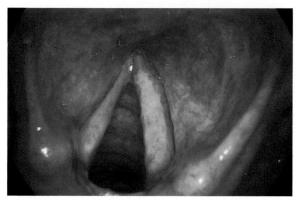

719

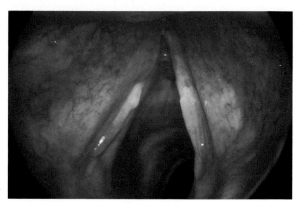

720

719 Leukoplakia of the larynx
The right vocal cord of this 74-year-old heavy cigarette smoker is markedly affected by the leukoplakia.

720 Leukoplakia with dysplasia of the vocal cords
There is leukoplakia of the middle thirds of both vocal cords in this 40-year-old heavy smoker. Histology showed leukoplakia with precancerous changes.

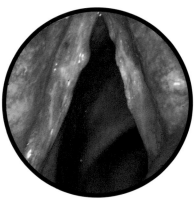

721

721 Chronic parakeratotic laryngitis
Thickening and irregularity of both cords are observed in this 47-year-old lawyer who had been hoarse for five years. He was a heavy smoker. The microscopic picture showed extensive dysplasia and atypical nuclei in the keratinized epithelial cells.

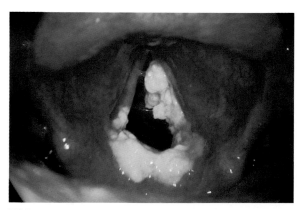

722

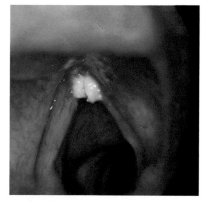

723

722 Hyperkeratosis of the larynx
The extensive hyperkeratotic lesions of the vocal cords and interarytenoid area proved, after excision of the whole lesion, not to be malignant.

723 Squamous cell carcinoma of the larynx
Clinically, this lesion in a 67-year-old male appeared to be a benign hyperkeratosis, such as the one seen in Fig. **722.** Histology showed this lesion to be a squamous cell carcinoma.

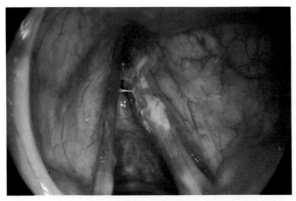

724

724 Carcinoma in situ of the right vocal cord
The whitish hyperplasia of the anterior portion of the right vocal cord proved to be carcinoma in situ on histology.

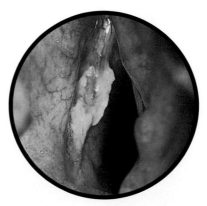

725

725 Carcinoma in situ of the left vocal cord
This lesion was decorticated from the vocal cord. Histology showed carcinoma in situ. The 75-year-old patient had been hoarse for two months.

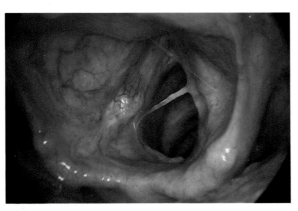

726

726 Squamous cell carcinoma of the left vocal cord
There is a circumscribed hyperplasia of the posterior half of the left vocal cord, and an irregular injection of the capillaries on the surface of the lesion. Histology showed invasive carcinoma. – There is a strand of mucous stretched across the glottis.

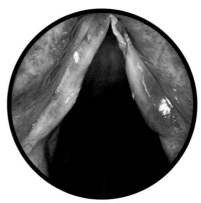

727

727 Squamous cell carcinoma of the right vocal cord
This 49-year-old patient was hoarse for two-and-one-half months. Both cords are edematous and leukoplakic. There is a whitish exudate on the ulcer on the most anterior portion of the right cord. Biopsy of this lesion showed carcinoma.

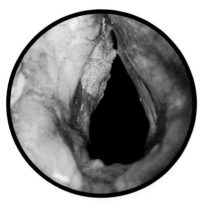

728

728 Carcinoma of the vocal cord
A carcinoma of the anterior half of the left vocal cord extending into the anterior commissure was observed in this 41-year-old woman. It was friable and verrucous and caused no motility impairment.

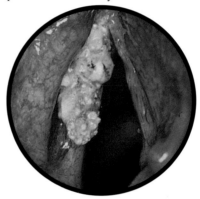

729

729 Carcinoma of the vocal cord
The patient was a 74-year-old woman with hoarseness of two months' duration. A superficial squamous cell carcinoma is seen on the superior and phonating surfaces of the midportion of the left vocal cord. No impairment of motility of the cord was noticed.

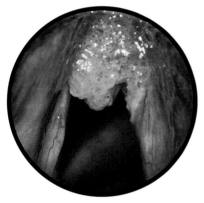

730

730 Carcinoma of the anterior glottis
The patient, a 56-year-old man, had been hoarse for four months. A papillary mass is seen to involve the anterior commissure and is invading the right vocal cord. The motility of the posterior half of the larynx was unimpaired, but the tumor prevented approximation of the cords anteriorly. Histologically it proved to be a verrucous carcinoma.

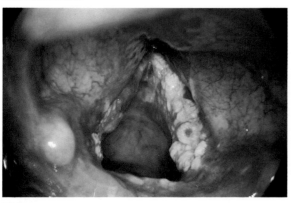

731

731 Verrucous carcinoma of the larynx
Carcinoma of the anterior two-thirds of the left vocal cord, the anterior commissure, and the anterior one-fourth of the right vocal cord of a man, 59 years of age.

732

732 Verrucous carcinoma of the glottis
There is a hyperkeratotic, ulcerated, hyperplastic lesion involving the entire glottis in this 41-year-old smoker. The motility of the right cord was limited.

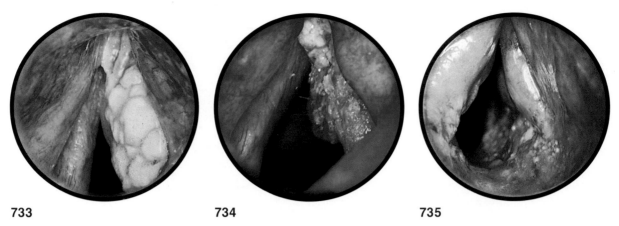

733   **734**   **735**

733 Carcinoma of the larynx
Moderately advanced carcinoma of the entire right vocal cord with invasion of the arytenoid as well as the anterior commissure. The right cord was fixed and the left cord showed keratotic involvement. The only complaint of this 67-year-old male was persistent, progressive hoarseness of six months' duration.

734 Squamous cell carcinoma of the vocal cord, right
The carcinoma involves the entire right cord and extends into the anterior commissure and into the right ventricle.

735 Subglottic carcinoma of the larynx
An extensive ulcerative subglottic carcinoma involves the right arytenoid area and fixes the right cord.

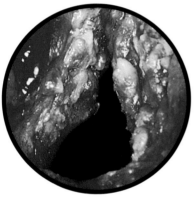

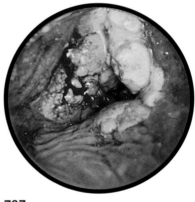

736   **737**

736 Transglottic carcinoma of the larynx
A circular glottic carcinoma observed in a 64-year-old male. In spite of the extent of this bilateral tumor, the motility of the cords was moderately good, suggesting that the lesion was relatively superficial or exophytic rather than invasive.

737 Advanced carcinoma of the larynx
A verrucous, ulcerative, circumferential carcinoma involving the entire larynx was demonstrated in a man 69 years of age with fixed bilateral cervical nodes. The tumor was friable and freely bleeding. It had almost totally obstructed the lumen of the glottis, leading to severe dyspnea in addition to hoarseness bordering on complete aphonia.

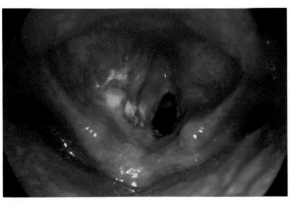

738 Secondary squamous cell carcinoma of the arytenoid, left
Fifteen years earlier, the patient had a frontolateral laryngectomy of the right side.

738

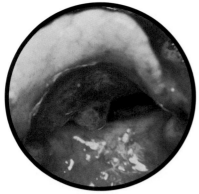

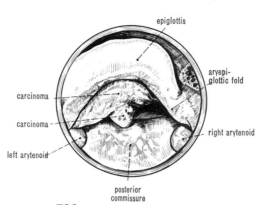

739

739a

739 Carcinoma of the epiglottis

Carcinoma of the laryngeal surface of the epiglottis. The laryngoscope tip has been placed in the vallecula, lifting the posterior surface into view. The tumor is broad-based, with a discrete projection in its midportion from which a biopsy sample of epidermoid carcinoma was obtained.

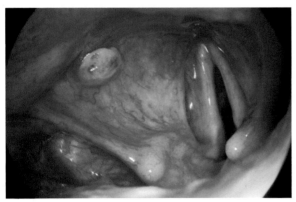

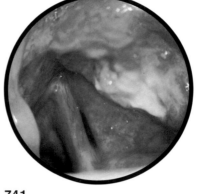

740

741

740 Early supraglottic squamous cell carcinoma of the laryngeal surface of the epiglottis

Lesions of the laryngeal surface of the epiglottis, such as this one and that in Fig. **739,** can be easily overlooked on mirror laryngoscopy. As shown here, the 90°-telescope exposes these lesions well.

741 Squamous cell carcinoma of the epiglottis

The angled telescope demonstrates the inferior extension of the lesion well. Since the glottis is not involved, a supraglottic partial laryngectomy is possible.

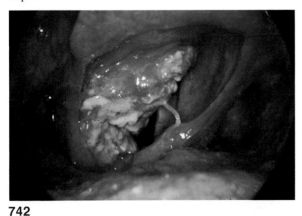

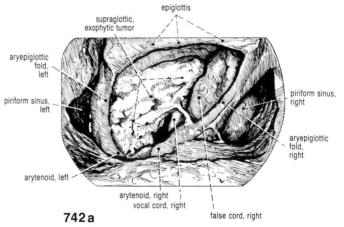

742

742a

742 Advanced squamous cell carcinoma of the larynx

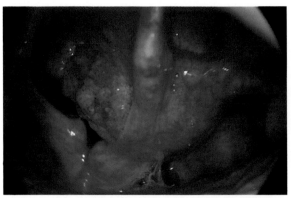

743

743 Squamous cell carcinoma of the supraglottic larynx
The tumor has spread through the right aryepiglottic fold into the piriform sinus.

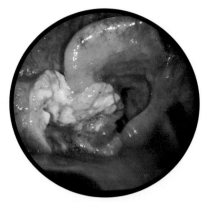

744

744 Squamous cell carcinoma of the aryepiglottic fold and piriform sinus
This extensive lesion involves the left piriform sinus, the aryepiglottic fold and left hemilarynx.

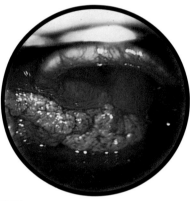

745

745 Postcricoid carcinoma
The arytenoids are edematous and the right arytenoid is

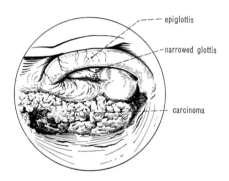

745a

fixed. The airway is markedly narrowed and the patient has severe dyspnea (mirror view). See Fig. **550.**

Uncommon Laryngeal Malignancies

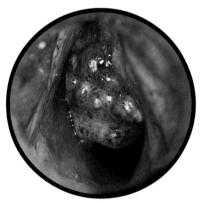

746

746 Carcinosarcoma of the larynx
This 85-year-old man noted persistent hoarseness of three months' duration and some difficulty in breathing during the ten days prior to examination.

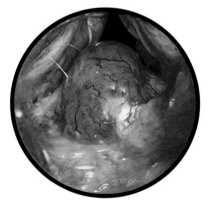

747

747 Malignant lymphoma of the larynx
A large rounded mass in the posterior commissure with infiltration of the subglottic tissues, caused severe respiratory obstruction in this 45-year-old woman.

Diseases of the Trachea and Bronchi

Diseases of the Trachea

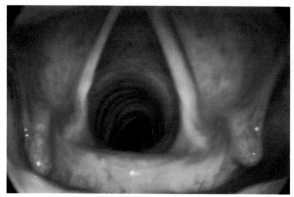

748

748　Normal trachea in the adult
The carina is faintly visible in this 90°-telescopic view.

Stenosis, Trauma and Inflammation

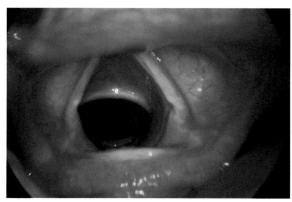

749

749　Subglottic space and trachea
This is a 90°-telescopic view of the prominent cricoid cartilage, the site of predilection of intubation injury and stenosis.

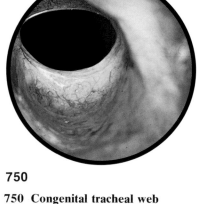

750

750　Congenital tracheal web
Web of the midtrachea in a 24-year-old man. He had always had slight dyspnea and occasionally an audible stridor.

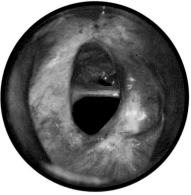

751

751　Stricture of the trachea
Tough fibrous stricture of the trachea at the level of the thoracic inlet in a 49-year-old woman with a persistent asthmatoid wheeze all her life.

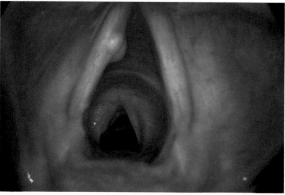

752

752　Tracheal stenosis
There is a tracheal stenosis which appears to be a second glottis at the site of a previous tracheotomy. There is a fibroma in the left vocal cord.

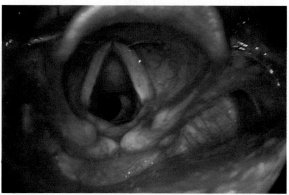

753

753 Tracheal stenosis, postintubation
There is a stenosis anteriorly at the cricoid level following long term intubation. Distally there is a second, half-moon stenotic lesion in the trachea (see Fig. **749**).

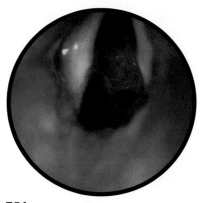

754

754 Severe subglottic stenosis
There is a severe anular subglottic stenosis with markedly narrowed airway. This lesion followed prolonged endotracheal intubation.

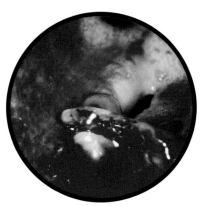

755

755 Traumatic tracheoesophageal fistula
Five days after an automobile accident in which this 19-year-old man's chest struck the steering wheel, he suddenly began to cough up liquid he had swallowed. An esophagogram showed a tracheoesophageal fistula in

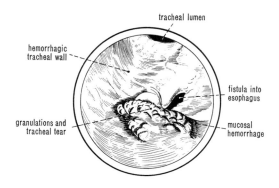

755 a

the midthoracic trachea. Tracheoscopy demonstrated an extensive hematoma on the posterior tracheal wall with granulations and a direct communication with the esophagus.

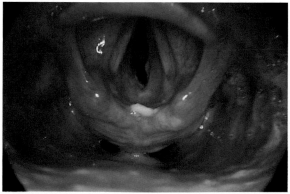

756

756 Stenosing laryngotracheitis sicca
The patient suffered severe attacks of pseudocroup.

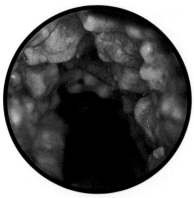

757

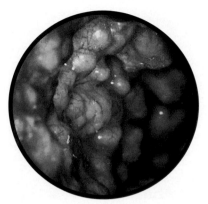

758

757–758 Tracheopathia osteoplastica
This 37-year-old female complained of cough, dyspnea, and occasional hemoptysis. – Fig. **757** shows glass hard protrusions which extended from the fourth tracheal ring to the carina. The calcifications were visible on a lateral x-ray of the trachea. – Fig. **758** is a view of the left tracheal wall.

Tumors

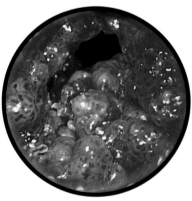

759

759 Papilloma of the trachea
This 59-year-old man complained of gradually increasing dyspnea and an asthmatoid wheeze associated with an uncontrollable cough. The chest radiogram was negative. The larynx was normal, but on tracheoscopy, a mass of papillomatous tissue was seen almost completely obstructing the thoracic trachea.

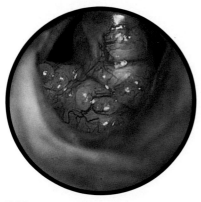

760

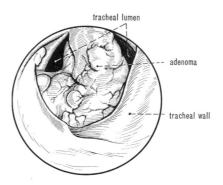

760 a

760 Subglottic adenoma

The patient was a 28-year-old woman who had developed severe stridor, dyspnea, and a constant irritating cough. Chest radiograms demonstrated bilateral emphysema. Numerous allergy surveys had been carried

out for three years because of what was considered to be an asthmatoid wheeze. An obstructing vascular tumor was found subglottically, originating from the posterior wall immediately below the level of the cords. Biopsy showed an adenoma of the carcinoid type.

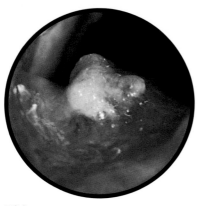

761

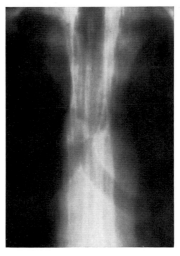

762

761–762 Adenocystic carcinoma of the trachea

A persistent productive cough that continued for four months developed in this 50-year-old woman. Occasional blood-streaked sputum, no chest pain. The tomogram disclosed a tumor on the right lateral tracheal

wall immediately above the orifice of the right main bronchus (Fig. **762**). Tracheoscopic examination revealed a soft, reddish, friable tumor covered with exudate on the floor and right lateral tracheal wall. Histology established the diagnosis.

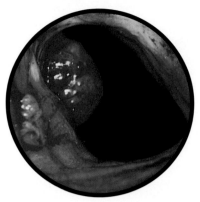

763

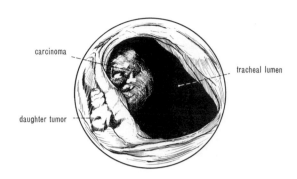

763a

763 Carcinoma of the trachea

A one-month history of cough, occasional hoarseness, and hemoptysis was elicited in this 48-year-old man. The vocal cords were found to be normal in configuration and motility on mirror examination, but blood was seen in the sputum in the posterior commissure, apparently arising from the trachea. The patient had stopped smoking ten years previously. Tomogram through the

upper trachea revealed a tumor on the left lateral tracheal wall at the level of the thoracic inlet. Visualized through the tracheoscope, this proved to be a lobulated circumscribed tumor with another tumor mass proximal to it. Histologic examination of the biopsy specimen demonstrates a poorly differentiated, infiltrating squamous cell carcinoma.

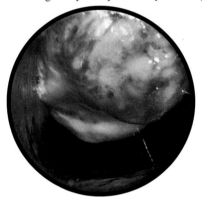

764

764 Fibrosarcoma of the trachea

This 76-year-old man was seen because of dyspnea, an audible stridor on both inspiration and expiration, a cough of two years' duration, and two episodes of severe hemoptysis. Tracheoscopy revealed a large soft tumor attached to the anterior tracheal wall. Biopsy proved it to be fibrosarcoma.

Diseases of the Bronchi

Endoscopic Anatomy

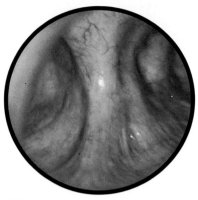

765

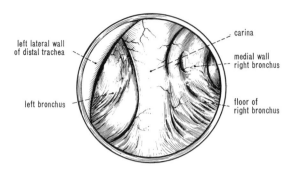

765a

765 The carina

The carina is seen as a prominent ridge (keel) dividing the trachea into the right and left bronchi. There may be considerable normal variation in the sharpness of its peak and the prominence of the cartilaginous pattern. In

this direct view, the right main bronchus is seen to descend 25 degrees from the midline; the left main bronchus branches at 75 degrees from the midline in monopodial diversion.

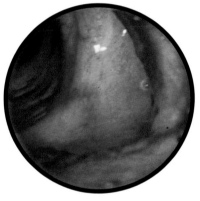

766

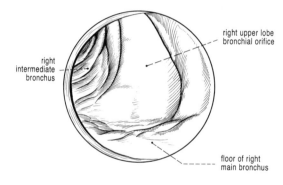

766a

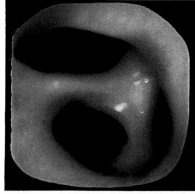

767

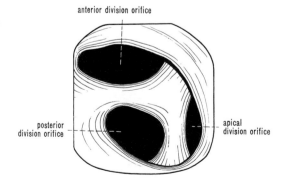

767a

766–767 The right upper lobe bronchus

The orifice of the upper lobe bronchus is seen as it originates from the lateral wall of the right main bronchus at a right angle to the axis of the main bronchus Fig. **766**. –

Fig. **767:** Telescopic (right-angle optic) view of the right upper lobe bronchus. The anterior, apical, and posterior segmental orifices are seen.

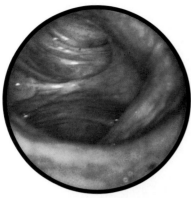

768

768a

768 The right middle lobe bronchus
The anterior wall of the right bronchus as it appears when looking directly into the middle lobe orifice. The lower lobe bronchus continues inferiorly.

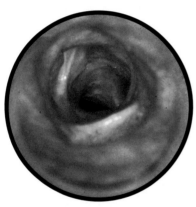

769

769a

769 The right lower lobe bronchus
Bronchoscopic view of the segmental orifices of the right lower lobe. With the lip of the bronchoscope just below the middle lobe orifice, the basilar branches as well as the superior division orifice are demonstrated.

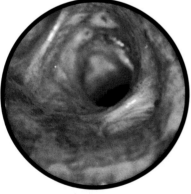

770

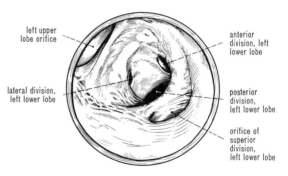

770a

770 The left bronchus
The left bronchus visualized from a point just proximal to the left upper lobe orifice. The upper lobe orifice is seen originating from the left anterolateral wall, the superior division of the left lower lobe on the posteromedial wall, and the anterior segmental orifice on the anteromedial wall. The posterior and lateral orifices are in shadow in the center of the field.

Bronchial Foreign Bodies

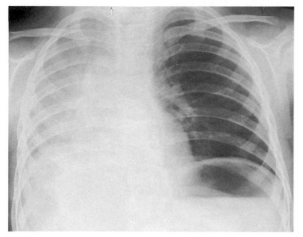

771

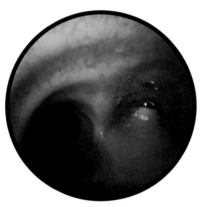

772

772a

771–772 Foreign body, right bronchus

For six weeks this two-year-old child was treated for bronchitis. Pediatric consultation revealed decreased breath sounds in the right lung. An x-ray, Fig. **771**, showed decreased aeration of the right lung and increased aeration on the left, mediastinal shift to the right and elevation of the right diaphragm, signs of obstructive atelectasis. Because of the right lung atelectasis, a bronchoscopy was done to rule out an obstructing foreign body or other cause for the bronchial stenosis. A peanut bathed in inflammatory exudate was found obstructing the right main bronchus, Fig. **772**. Peanuts are a common and dangerous foreign body aspirated into the lungs of children. Radiologic or clinical findings of bronchial stenosis such as seen here are an indication for bronchoscopy to diagnose and correct the bronchial obstruction.

anterior tracheal wall

peanut

secretion

carina

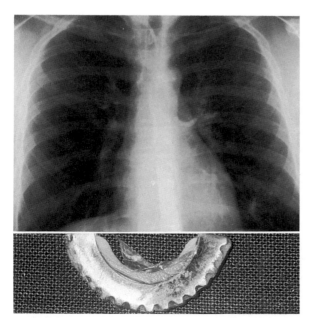

773

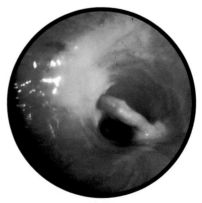

774

773–774 Foreign body, metal toy, left bronchus

The x-ray, Fig. **773**, shows a portion of a bird whistle in the left main bronchus. At bronchoscopy, Fig. **774**, the encrusted edge of the foreign body is seen lodged in the left main bronchus. The extracted foreign body is seen in the inset of Fig. **773**.

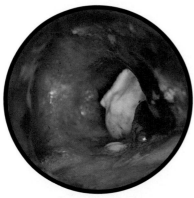

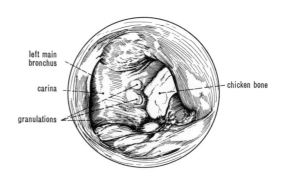

775

775a

775 Foreign body, right bronchus
Fragment of chicken bone, right main and intermediate bronchi. Frequent spasms of coughing, wheezing, and occasional hemoptysis had occurred for three months.

The history of "choking" on a chicken bone was obtained prior to this examination. Friable granulations surround the impacted bone.

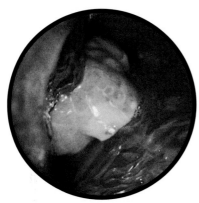

776

776 Foreign body, left main bronchus
A 21-year-old female complained of pain in the left side of the chest, dyspnea, cough, unilateral wheezing, and occasional hemoptysis. She recalled a severe episode of coughing while eating chicken five years previously. The bronchoscopic examination showed inflammation of the left main bronchus with granulation tissues partially occluding the lumen. The chicken bone was transfixed across the lumen, buried in the soft friable granulations.

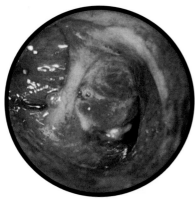

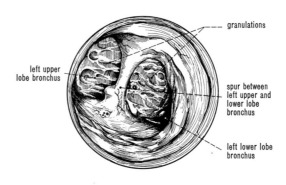

777

777a

777 Foreign body, left bronchus
A 47-year-old man had been treated for chronic pulmonary disease. He had aspirated a collar button at 10 years of age. Parts of the button were still visible on the radiogram and endoscopically were seen to have eroded through the spur between the left lower and upper lobe

bronchi. There were extensive bronchiectatic changes in both upper and lower lobes. Distortion and fibrous granulation tissue changes of the orifices of the upper and lower lobe bronchi are observed. The bronchial spur between them can be identified.

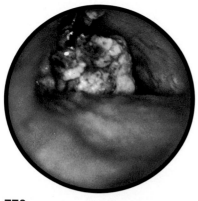

778

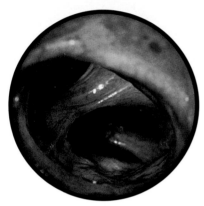

779

779 Anthracosis
Pigment discoloring the mucosa of the left upper and left

778 Broncholithiasis
Broncholith in the right lower lobe bronchus. This endogenous foreign body has many sharp irregular projections that hold it firmly fixed in the bronchial lumen.

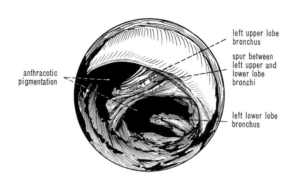

779a

lower lobe bronchi of a coal miner. The right side was likewise involved.

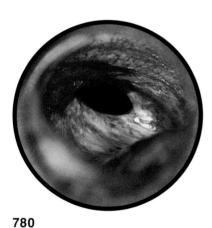

780

780 Cicatricial bronchial stenosis
Benign stenosis of the right intermediate bronchus in this 32-year-old man followed rupture of the bronchus resulting from an automobile accident. Primary repair of the bronchus by end-to-end anastomosis was followed by periodic dilatations.

Inflammatory Diseases

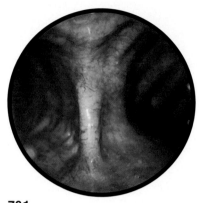

781

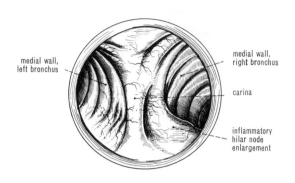

781a

781 Bronchitis
In this 36-year-old man who was exposed to smoke in a burning building, the inflammatory changes consist of a

reddened mucosa, prominence of the vascular pattern, and hilar node enlargement.

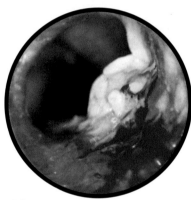

782

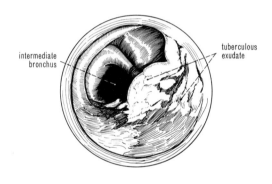

782a

782 Endobronchial tuberculosis
Ulcerative, exudate-covered tuberculous granuloma of the right upper lobe bronchus. The ulceration extends upward along the lateral wall of the right main bronchus

and the trachea. The inflammatory reaction of the entire mucosal surface and the soft granular appearance of the mucosa suggest an inflammatory rather than a neoplastic process.

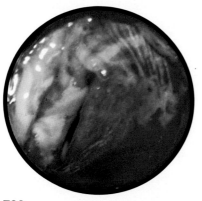

783

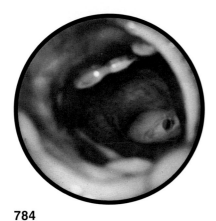

784

783 Endobronchial tuberculosis
Diffuse mucosal involvement by tuberculosis of the lat-

783 a

eral and anterior walls of the left main bronchus. The caseous tuberculous exudate is typical of this disease.

784 Bronchiectasis
Bronchoscopic appearance of viscid purulent secretions adherent to the bronchial walls in a patient with chronic bronchiectasis.

Middle Lobe Syndrome

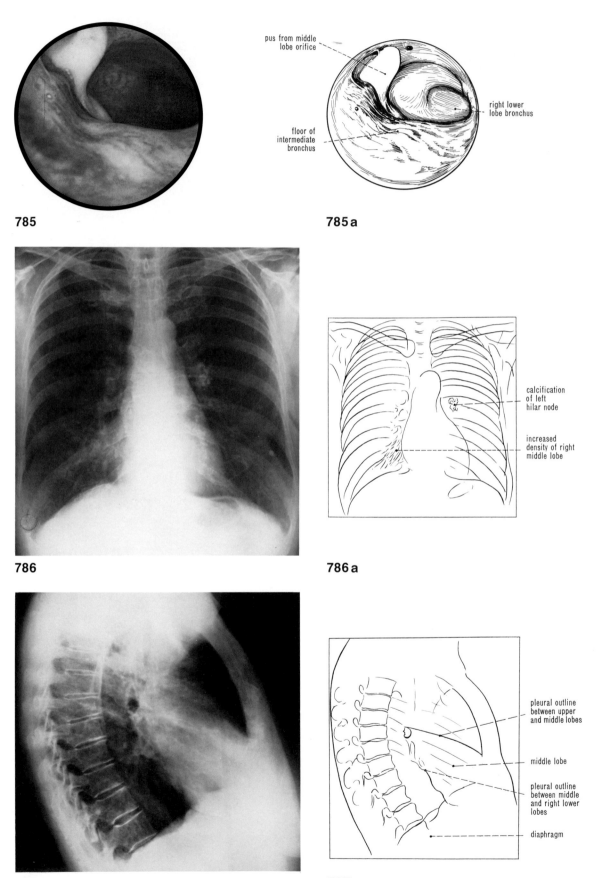

785

785a

pus from middle
lobe orifice

right lower
lobe bronchus

floor of
intermediate
bronchus

786

786a

calcification
of left
hilar node

increased
density of right
middle lobe

787

787a

pleural outline
between upper
and middle lobes

middle lobe

pleural outline
between middle
and right lower
lobes

diaphragm

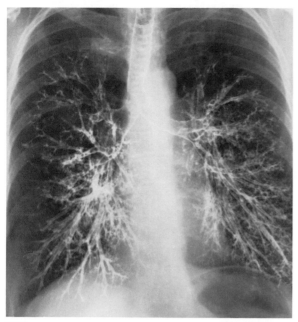

788

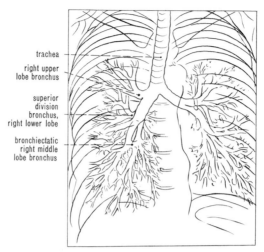

788a

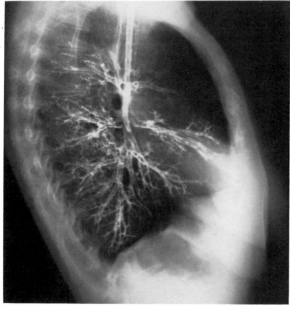

789

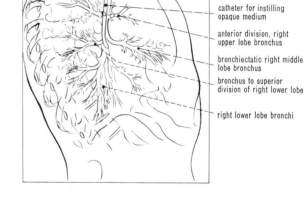

789a

785–789 Middle lobe syndrome

The middle lobe syndrome is the result of acute or chronic infiltration, contraction or atelectasis of the middle lobe. Various lesions may cause the syndrome, such as bronchogenic carcinoma, bronchial tuberculosis and compression of the middle lobe bronchus by tuberculosis, malignant lymphoma or lymph node metastases. The patient, a woman 38 year of age, had a productive cough, occasional episodes of hemoptysis, and recurring attacks of right-sided "pneumonia." Purulent secretions are seen exuding from the stenotic orifice of the middle

lobe, Fig. **785**. Figs. **786–787**: Posteroanterior and lateral chest radiograms indicate an infiltrate in the region of the right middle lobe, characteristic of the middle lobe syndrome. Fig. **788**: The posteroanterior bronchogram demonstrates a normal configuration of the tracheobronchial tree except for the cluster of bronchi superimposed on each other extending inferiorly from the right hilum. The lateral bronchogram, Fig. **789**, discloses cylindrical dilation of the middle lobe bronchi, which are crowded together in the atelectatic right middle lobe.

Bronchial Tumors

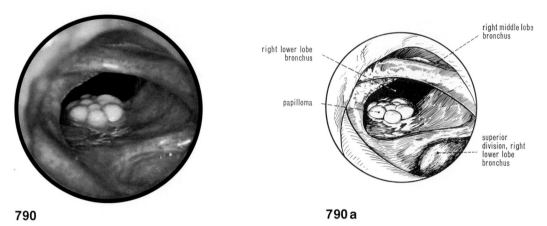

790

790a

790 Papilloma of the bronchus
Incidental finding of an isolated asymptomatic papilloma on the floor of the right lower lobe bronchus.

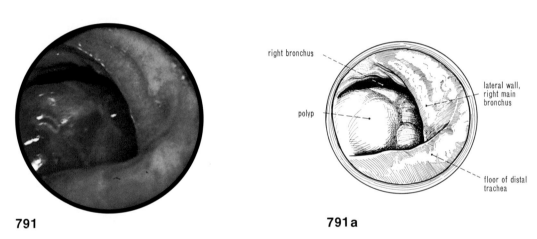

791

791a

791 Polyp of the bronchus
Large pedunculated polyp at the entrance of the right bronchus. The to-and-fro motion during respiration produced obstructive emphysema of the right lung.

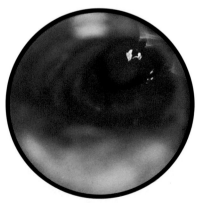

792

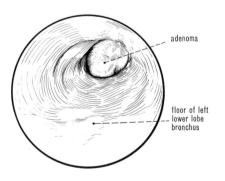

792a

792 Bronchial adenoma, left lower lobe bronchus
This 34-year-old woman had a history of repeated episodes of pleurisy and pneumonia in the left lower chest, posteriorly. Chest radiograms revealed atelectasis of the basilar segment of the left lower lobe. The smooth round tumor obstructing the segmental bronchus bled readily. Histologic study confirmed the clinical impression of a bronchial adenoma.

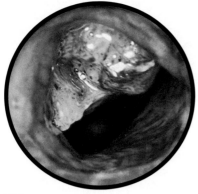

793

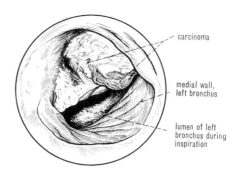

793a

793 Bronchogenic carcinoma

This 66-year-old man was referred because of weight loss, dyspnea, and cough. Obstructive emphysema of the entire left lung was found on physical examination and

confirmed by radiograms. Bronchoscopic study disclosed a friable verrucous tumor, partially obstructing the left bronchus on inspiration and completely obstructing it during expiration.

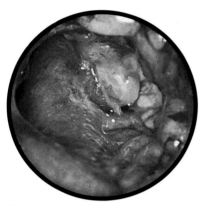

794

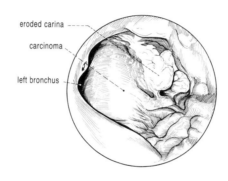

794a

794 Bronchogenic carcinoma

Severe dyspnea and acute pneumonic symptoms affecting the left lung were present in this 61-year-old man. A chest roentgenogram showed a pleural effusion, and after drainage, a mass was noted in the left hilus. Bron-

choscopic examination demonstrated a tumor occluding the left main bronchus, eroding the carina, and extending upward along the floor of the distral trachea. Biopsy proved it to be an anaplastic, poorly differentiated (oat cell) carcinoma.

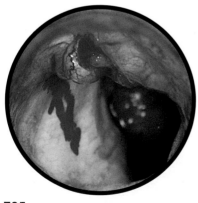

795

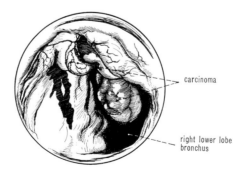

795a

795 Bronchogenic carcinoma

Carcinoma of the middle and right lower lobe bronchi. The tumor is seen to extrude from the middle lobe

orifice as a somewhat friable, vascular, rounded mass. It extends downward to partially obstruct the right lower lobe bronchus.

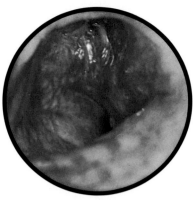

796

796 Bronchogenic carcinoma
View of the right main stem bronchus showing a bronchogenic carcinoma originating in the middle lobe. The

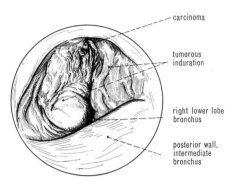

796a

middle lobe orifice is occluded, and edema and induration involve the entrance to the right lower lobe bronchus.

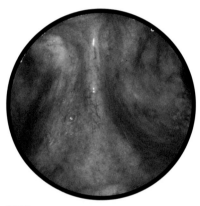

797

797 The broad carina
Nodular appearance of the carina, suggesting mediastinal metastatic disease. The patient was a 61-year-old man whose radiogram showed left hilar thickening. The

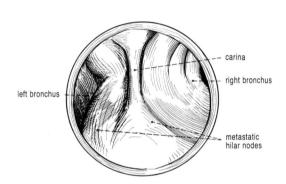

797a

bronchoscopic examination otherwise was essentially negative, but tumor cells were found in washings of the left bronchus.

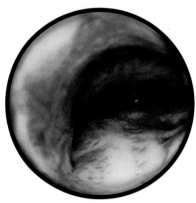

798

798 Bronchial invasion by esophageal carcinoma
Invasion of the right main bronchus by direct extension of a carcinoma from the midthoracic esophagus.

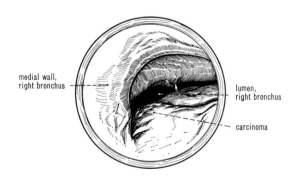

798a

Diseases
of the Esophagus

Endoscopic Anatomy

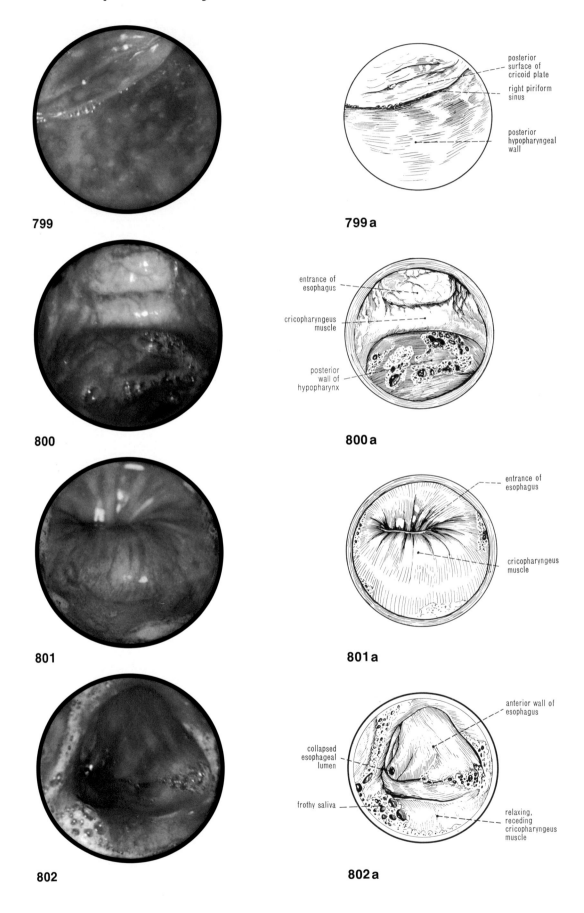

799

799 a
- posterior surface of cricoid plate
- right piriform sinus
- posterior hypopharyngeal wall

800

800 a
- entrance of esophagus
- cricopharyngeus muscle
- posterior wall of hypopharynx

801

801 a
- entrance of esophagus
- cricopharyngeus muscle

802

802 a
- anterior wall of esophagus
- collapsed esophageal lumen
- frothy saliva
- relaxing, receding cricopharyngeus muscle

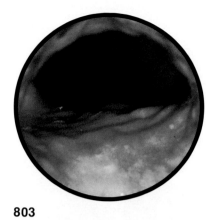

803

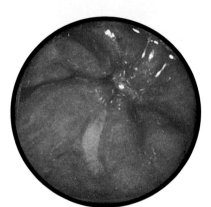

804

804 The cardia
Esophagoscopically, the cardia is seen as a sphincter

803 The normal thoracic esophagus
The esophageal lumen remains patent during quiet respiration when the esophagoscope is in place. A small rippling contraction wave is observed preceding the esophagoscope as it advances through the thoracic esophagus.

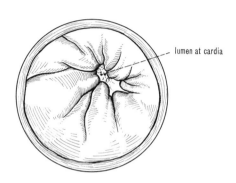

lumen at cardia

804 a

with rolled puckered edges meeting in a point that indicates the lumen into the stomach.

◀ **799–802 Introduction of the rigid esophagoscope**
First step (Fig. 799): With the patient supine the esophagoscope is introduced into the hypopharynx to the right of the midline and advanced with anterior guidance into the right piriform sinus. This view shows the posterior surface of the cricoid plate anteriorly and the posterior wall of the hypopharynx posteriorly.

800 Second step. The larynx is lifted forward by the lip of the advancing esophagoscope to reveal the entrance of the esophagus, which remains closed by the contracted cricopharyngeus muscle. The esophageal entrance is seen as a slitlike opening anteriorly with the edge of the muscle in the center of the field. The most common site of perforation occurring during esophagos-

copy is the posterior half of the field, below the edge of the cricopharyngeus muscle when the instrument is forcibly driven through the posterior wall of the hypopharynx into the superior mediastinal space.

801 Third step: After slight hesitation, the cricopharyngeus relaxes and begins to fall posteriorly to reveal more clearly the esophageal entrance.

802 Fourth step: The mucosal lining of the cervical esophagus. The lumen remains closed until after the open esophagoscope passes the cricopharyngeus when the negative intrathoracic pressure of the first inspiration allows it to expand.

Inflammation, Chemical Burns, and Strictures

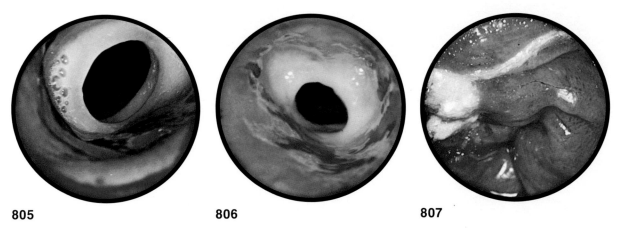

805   806   807

805 Congenital esophageal web
This 15-year-old boy had been considered a "feeding problem" because of slow eating habits and refusal to eat solids. He had several episodes of foreign body lodgment in the esophagus but had been able to expel the objects spontaneously. Esophagrams demonstrated this web at the level of the thoracic inlet following esophagoscopic removal of an impacted piece of sausage.

806 Lye stricture of the esophagus
Stricture of the esophagus of a 24-year-old woman who had accidentally ingested lye in childhood. The scar is spiral rather than circular, and the edges are firm and avascular.

807 Acute esophagitis
Diffuse esophagitis in a 48-year-old woman who complained of substernal pain, burning, and dysphagia. Edema, redness, excessive secretions, and exudate characterize the condition.

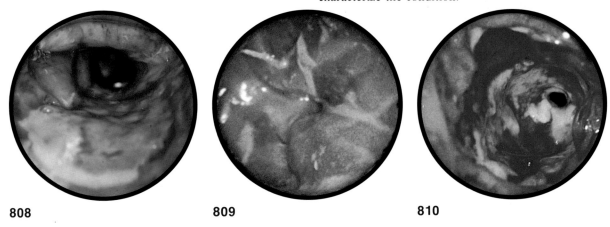

808   809   810

808 Fresh lye burn of the esophagus

809 Fresh hydrochloric acid burn of the esophagus

810 Peptic esophagitis
Severe ulcerative esophagitis with a rigid stricture of the cardia. The stricture remains patent, allowing gastric secretion to flow back and forth to produce a reflux esophagitis.

Foreign Bodies

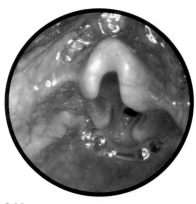

812

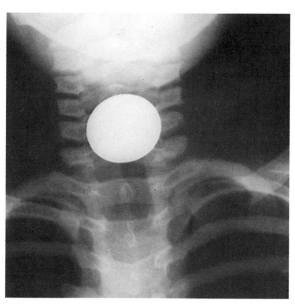

811

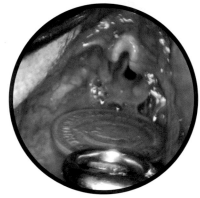

813

811–813 Foreign body, coin, in the cervical esophagus
Coins are perhaps the most common foreign body occurring in children. – Fig. **811** is the x-ray view of the coin. –

Fig. **812** shows the telescopic view of the coin. The upper rim of the coin is just visible in the postcricoid region. – Fig. **813** shows removal of the foreign body.

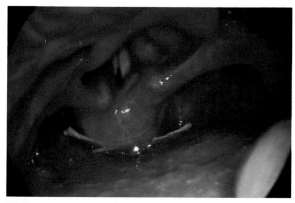

814

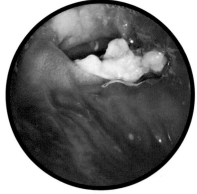

815

814 Foreign body, bone, hypopharynx
The bone lies across the postcricoid region.

815 Foreign body, chicken bone, cervical esophagus
The chicken bone lies just below the fold of the cricopharyngeus muscle.

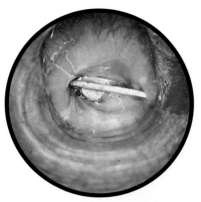

816

816 Foreign body, toy key, in cervical esophagus
The key lies in the cervical esophagus of a two-year-old.

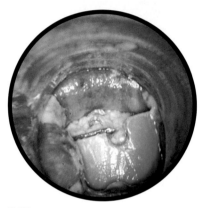

817

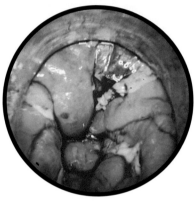

818

817–818 Foreign body, cervical esophagus
This 19-year-old patient swallowed a pencil sharpener nine days earlier. An attempt to remove the foreign body failed. Esophagoscopy, Fig. **817**, shows the blue foreign body and a fibrinous ulceration of the esophageal mucosa caused by the sharp edge of the pen-

cil sharpener. There are traces of ingested food caught by the foreign body. In Fig. **818** the inflammation caused by the previous attempts at removal and the prolonged sojourn of the foreign body is seen. There are edema, membranous ulceration, and traces of blood.

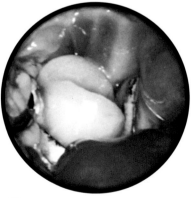

819

819 Foreign body in the esophagus
A removable, single-tooth prosthesis was impacted in the cervical esophagus for five days. Traumatic edema of the mucosa is apparent. The metal hooks that should have held it to adjacent teeth can be seen embedded in the mucosa.

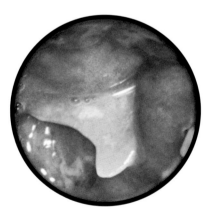

820 Foreign body, dental prosthesis, cervical esophagus
There is a broken portion of a dental plate lodged in the cervical esophagus. The tip of the posterior edge of the plate is seen as the esophagoscope approaches the foreign body. There is traumatic mucosal edema.

Diverticula

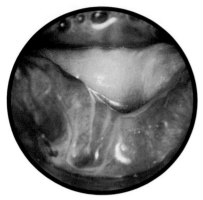

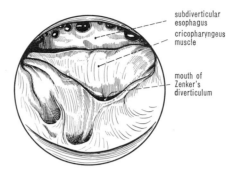

821

821a

821 Zenker's diverticulum

A 79-year-old man with dysphagia noted gurgling when swallowing, regurgitation of small quantities of undigested food, and constant cough. Radiograms demonstrated a characteristic hypopharyngeal pulsion diver-

ticulum. The esophageal speculum has lifted the cricoid plate anteriorly to expose the cricopharyngeus muscle transversely across the lumen as it separates the entrance to the diverticulum, seen posteriorly, from the subdiverticular esophagus, anteriorly.

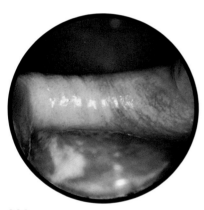

822

822 Zenker's diverticulum

Slotted esophagoscope with the anterior blade introduced into the subdiverticular esophagus and the posterior blade into the diverticulum. The cricopharyngeus is engaged between the two blades.

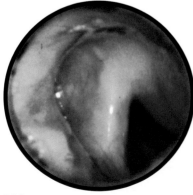

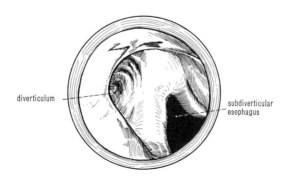

823

823a

823 Traction diverticulum

This diverticulum was found in a 62-year-old woman who complained of dysphagia, precordial pain, and pain radiating to the back between the scapulas during swal-

lowing. – The wide open mouth of the diverticulum lies to the left of the photo and the esophageal lumen to the right. A barium x-ray study demonstrated the lesion in the thoracic esophagus.

Fistulas and Trauma

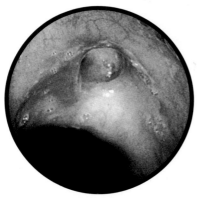

824

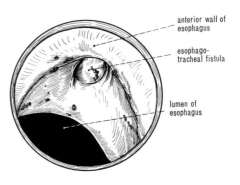

824 a

824 Tracheoesophageal fistula

Esophagoscopic appearance of a fistulous tract entrance in the anterior wall of the midthoracic esophagus. The patient was a 64-year-old man with a constant productive cough of two years' duration, loss of weight, and recurrent episodes of pneumonia. His cough was most persistent during meals and was especially aggravated when he was swallowing fluids. The entrance of the tract into the medial wall of the left main bronchus was discovered. Subsequent surgical resection revealed a calcified hilar node adherent to both the bronchial and esophageal walls.

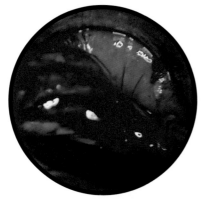

825

825 Acute perforation of the middle third of the esophagus following introduction of a flexible gastroscope

This perforation was confirmed by a lipiodal swallow radiograph. The mediastinum is seen through the inflamed and hemorrhagic perforation in the lower part of the photo. In the upper portion of the photo the esophageal lumen is visible. Within the lumen there is a metal aspirator at 4 o'clock in the photo.

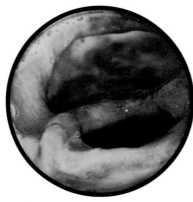

826

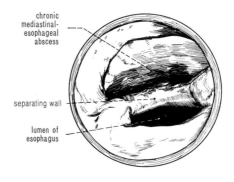

826 a

826 Chronic esophageal perforation and mediastinal abscess

This 58-year-old man had had a right-sided empyema and intermittent bouts of pulmonary infection for two years. Food would appear occasionally in the empyema drainage, and he had lost 36 pounds. A history was obtained of "choking" on a chicken bone before the onset of symptoms. Esophagoscopic examination shows a large esophageal perforation anteriorly, leading into a well walled-off anterior mediastinal abscess. The abscess had drained into the right pleural cavity, which was subsequently drained through the right chest wall. The esophagus is the elliptical lumen in the posterior half of the field.

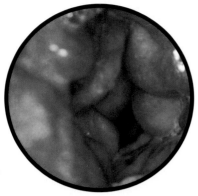

827

827 Esophageal varices
Multiple large esophageal varices as they are seen involving the entire circumference of the walls of the distal esophagus. The varices extended from the cervical esophagus to the cardia. There is no complicating esophagitis.

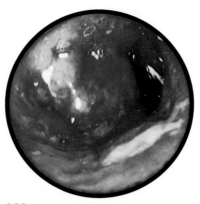

828

828 Hilar node invasion of the esophagus
Dysphagia and substernal pain were the chief complaints of this 46-year-old female. The chest radiogram revealed an irregular calcified mass in the right hilus, and the esophagogram showed that the mass compressed the esophagus, as confirmed by the esophagoscopic examination. On subsequent surgical exploration, a large inflammatory, irregular, partially calcified mass was found, probably the result of histoplasmosis.

Tumors

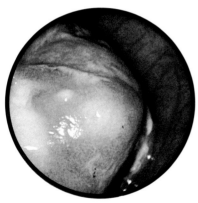

829

829 Multiple pedunculated fibromas of the esophagus
This 48-year-old man became nauseated and vomited a mass which he realized remained attached deep in the throat and which he could not expel. The radiogram demonstrated a number of irregular filling defects involving the full length of the esophageal lumen. On esophagoscopic examination these smooth, round, intraluminal masses appeared; they proved to be fibromas.

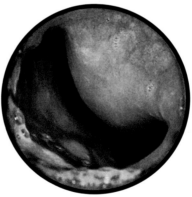

830

830 Leiomyoma of the esophagus
Submucosal tumor compressing the right anterolateral wall of the midthoracic esophagus. The patient was a 60-year-old male who had moderate dysphagia and intermittent substernal discomfort. The diagnosis of leiomyoma was confirmed by thoracotomy and resection of the tumor. Esophagoscopic biopsy of the mucosa was not performed, and the lumen of the esophagus was not entered during the thoracotomy.

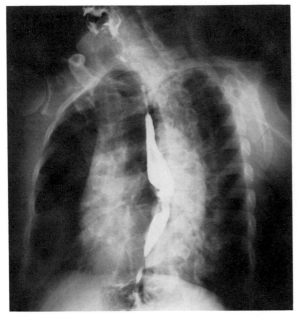

831

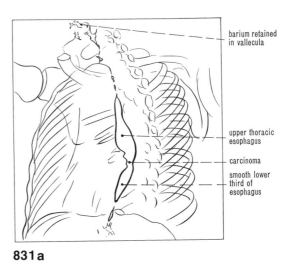

831a

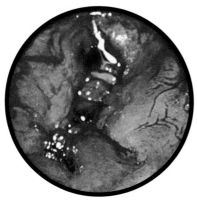

832

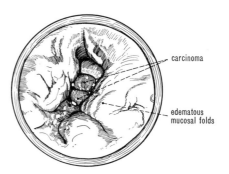

832a

831–832 Carcinoma of the esophagus

The patient was a 74-year-old male who experienced increasing dysphagia over a period of six months. The radiogram demonstrates an irregular filling defect and stenosis of the esophagus at the junction of its middle and lower thirds (Fig. **831**). On esophagoscopic examination a friable mass was found in the stenotic lumen, (Fig. **832**). Biopsy proved it to be a nonkeratinizing squamous cell carcinoma.

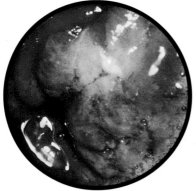

833

833 Carcinoma of the esophagus

This 67-year-old male complained for several months of dysphagia, cough, chest pains and weight loss. Esophagoscopy showed this large, fungating, easily bleeding lesion in the upper thoracic esophagus.

Diseases
of the Neck

Congenital Anomalies

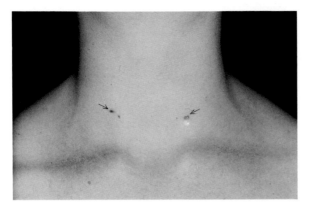

834

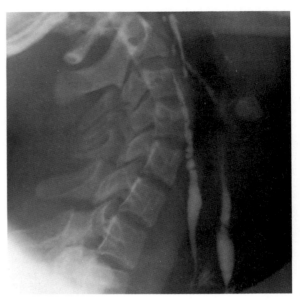

835

834–835 Lateral fistulas of the neck
Neck fistulas and sinuses arise from persistent cervical sinuses and cervicobranchial ducts. The openings of the fistulas arise from the second, third or fourth branchial arches and occur at different levels of the neck anterior to the sternocleidomastoid muscle between the clavicle and the mandible. The 18-year-old patient in Fig. **834**

has two fistulas at the neck root. In Fig. **835** contrast medium has been injected into the fistulas seen in Fig. **834**. The radiograph shows that the fistulous tracts reach to the supratonsillar fossae. This case is an example of complete lateral neck fistulas in which there is a direct connection from the endodermal pharynx to the ectodermal skin of the neck.

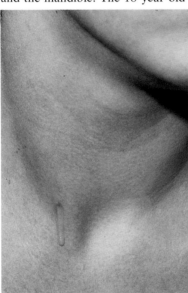

836

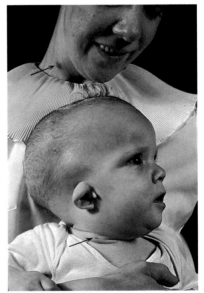

837

836 Lateral neck fistula
Bacterial infection of neck fistulas is common. As seen here, there is pus exuding from this infected lesion. The cranialward course of the tract appears as a fibrous strand beneath the skin overlying the sternocleidomastoid muscle.

837 Congenital cervical fistulas
Hereditary patterns of development of the first branchial arch are demonstrated by this mother and her 4-month-old infant, both of whom have branchial cleft sinuses at the anterior borders of the sternocleidomastoid muscles, arrows. The child also has bilateral microtia and polyotia.

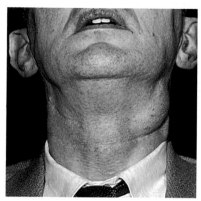

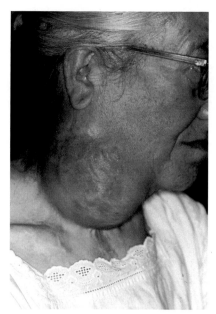

838

839

838–839 Lateral cysts of the neck
These cysts probably originate from the cervical sinus. Recently their branchiogenic origin has been questioned. They occur at different levels, generally anterior to the sternocleidomastoid muscle, Fig. **838**. They can lie beneath the muscle. Their size varies and at times

reach extremely large size, as in this 70-year-old patient, Fig. **839**. – The cysts usually fluctuate. The diagnosis of a branchial cleft cyst carcinoma should be made with greatest caution, since most malignant tumors of the neck represent lymphogenous or hematogenous metastases from an occult or undiagnosed primary lesion.

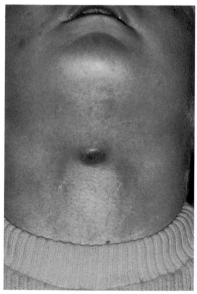

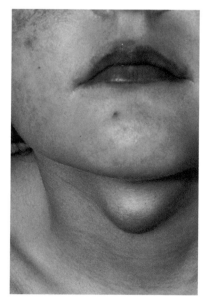

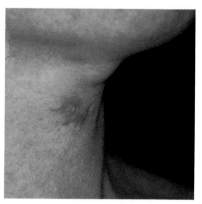

840   **841**   **842**

840–842 Thyroglossal duct cysts and fistulas
Midline neck fistulas, Fig. **840** and cysts, Fig. **841**, are embryologic remnants of the thyroglossal duct which developed as a pouch from the foramen cecum on the tongue to the thyroid gland. The cysts and fistulas move

with swallowing. The epithelium of the cysts and fistulas is intricately related to the body of the hyoid bone. Recurrent cysts and fistulas, Fig. **842** occur when the entire cyst including the body of the hyoid are not removed at surgery. The recurrent cyst lies above the surgical scar.

Specific and Nonspecific Inflammation

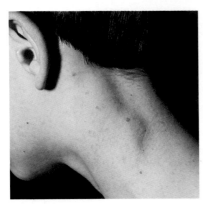

843

843 Lymph node swelling with German measles
This lymph node enlargement is typical for that which is associated with German measles and occurred in an 18-year-old male. Without the exanthem, or other symptoms of upper respiratory involvement, toxoplasmosis, tuberculosis, nasopharyngeal carcinoma or malignant lymphoma would have to be ruled out with lymph node enlargement such as this.

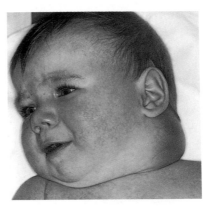

844

844 Cervical lymphadenitis, nonspecific
Cervical lymphadenitis, as seen here, is common in children and follows streptococcus or staphylococcus infections of the mouth and throat. A Bezold's mastoid abscess should be ruled out by an otoscopic examination.

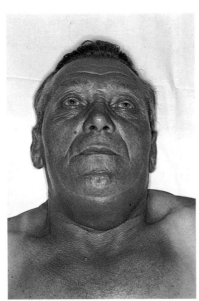

845

845 Phlegmon of the neck; Angina Ludovici
Abscess and brawny infiltration followed extraction of two lower molar teeth.

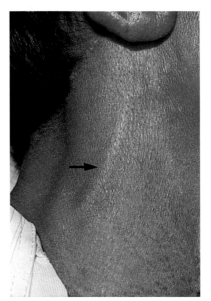

846

846 Auricular nerve involvement in lepromatous leprosy
The greater auricular nerve is enlarged by leprous infiltration of the perineurium. The leprous involvement of the auricle appears in the upper photo. The peroneal and ulnar nerve are also characteristically involved in leprosy. See also Figs **38, 373**.

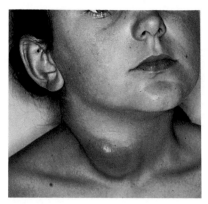

847

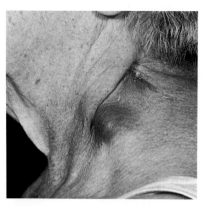

848

847 Cervical lymph node tuberculosis
This Balkan native suffers from three stages of tuberculosis. 1) tuberculous cervical lymphadenitis, 2) spread of tuberculosis to the perinodal soft tissues of the neck and 3) tuberculosis of the skin. The primary lesion in the tonsil healed and the lungs are clear. This is an example of ingestion tuberculosis which seldom occurs where bovine tuberculosis has been eliminated. A conservative neck dissection was done and the tubercle bacilli were found in the biopsy.

848 Tuberculous lymph nodes
Fig. **848** shows a 75-year-old woman who stated that she had enlarged nodes of the neck in childhood. An old retracted scar at the hairline resulted from specific fistulous lymph node suppuration. The patient had a fluctuant lateral cervical lymph node with infiltration into the dermis. A radiogram of the chest showed old specific areas of infection in both apices. Following extirpation, the histological picture was that of caseating tuberculous lymphadenitis with specific involvement of the skin. Seemingly inactive, old specific foci in the lung may spread through blood channels into peripheral lymph nodes in cases in which the resistance of the patient has been disturbed. Exacerbation of an old focus is possible after years, even decades, in patients with primary lymphogenic infiltrated tuberculous neck nodes.

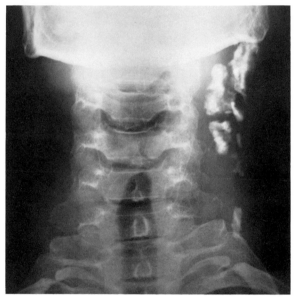

849

849 Tuberculosis, cervical lymph nodes
The radiogram of the neck shows extensive calcified lymphadenopathy on the left, typical of scrofula.

Tumors

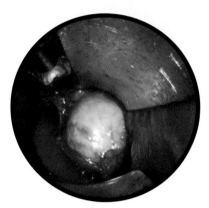

850

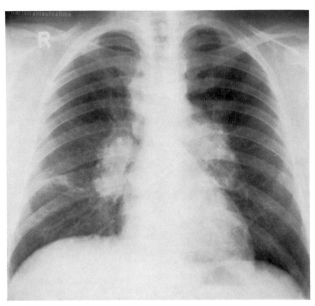

851

850–851 Sarcoidosis

This systemic disease (Besnier-Boeck-Schaumann syndrome) may affect every tissue and organ in the body. Lymph nodes, spleen, lung, liver, bone, tonsils, skin, as well as eyes, lacrimal and salivary glands (uveoparotid fever of Heerfordt), and other structures in the head and neck region may be involved. Prescalene node biopsy and mediastinoscopy with lymph node biopsy aid in the diagnosis. Fig. **850** shows a rounded sarcoid lymph node in the left tracheobronchial angle exposed at mediastinoscopy. The grayish white, occasionally bluish red appearance and fleshy consistency of the lymph nodes coupled with the lack of adhesions and the increase in capillary bleeding are typical. The left lateral wall of the trachea is seen on the right. The frontal radiogram of the chest shows bilateral hilar and upper mediastinal adenopathy. In addition some fine parenchymal infiltration is noted in the right midlung field (Fig. **851**).

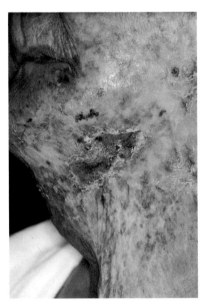

852

852 Carcinoma superimposed on lupus vulgaris

Carcinoma occurs frequently in old scarred lupus vulgaris lesions. This lesion occurred in a lupus lesion that was previously treated with x-ray.

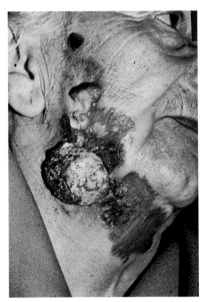

853

853 Squamous cell carcinoma and lupus vulgaris

There is an exophytic carcinoma that has arisen in an active lupus vulgaris field.

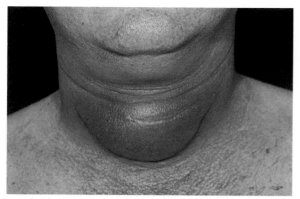

854

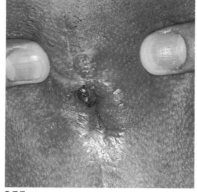

855

854 Midline abscess of the neck

Six weeks prior to this photograph, a horizontal incision was made for a laryngofissure for carcinoma involving the anterior commissure. The superficial secondary infection is seen here. Such complications following thyrotomy arouse suspicion of a persistent tumor or the possibility of skin seeding (see also Fig. **855**).

855 Persistent laryngeal carcinoma postlaryngofissure and cordectomy

An incompletely removed carcinoma has penetrated through the laryngofissure incision to the surface of the neck.

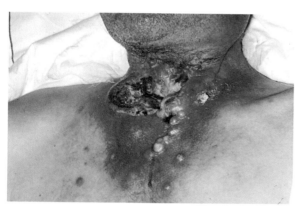

856

856 Subglottic carcinoma with recurrence

A laryngectomy and bilateral neck dissection followed by x-ray therapy were performed in this 60-year-old male. There were lymph node metastases in the peritracheal chain which could not be removed surgically. The recurrent tumor has infiltrated externally around the tracheal stoma. An indication of the malignancy of the lesion and the lowered immunologic resistance of the patient is seen in the nodular metastases in the chest skin. Recurrent hemoptysis signalled the eventual fatal outcome from arrosion of the common carotid artery.

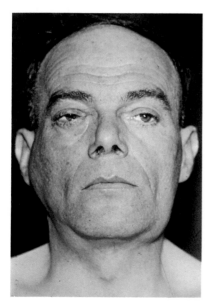

857

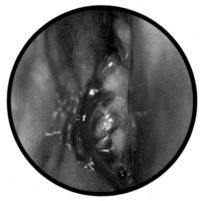

858

857–858 Metastasizing ethmoid squamous cell carcinoma

This patient has a narrowed right palpebral fissure and hard, nodular enlargments of the right parotid and both submaxillary gland regions, Fig. **857**. – Nasal endoscopy, Fig. **858**, shows a nodular carcinomatous lesion in the superior nasal vault, which arose from the ethmoid sinuses on the right. The nasal septum is on the right side of the photo (see also Figs. **459–461**).

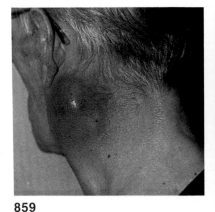

859

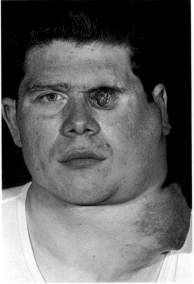

860

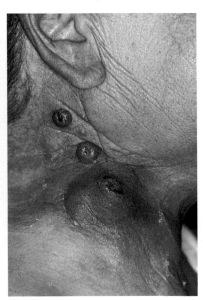

861

859 Nasopharyngeal carcinoma with superior cervical metastases
High cervical lymph node metastases under the superior attachment of the sternocleidomastoid muscle are often as in this case the first sign of a clinically silent malignancy of the nasopharynx. See Figs **496–498**.

860 Metastatic melanoma from the choroid
This 33-year-old male had undergone exenteration of the orbit for a choroidal melanoma two years previously.

At the time this photograph was taken there were extensive metastases to the parotid, submandibular and lateral cervical regions.

861 Metastatic carcinoma from the base of the tongue
The patient had undergone surgery and irradiation of the primary lesion in the tongue and neck. In spite of this, the condition progressed to involvement and ulceration of the skin and neck nodes.

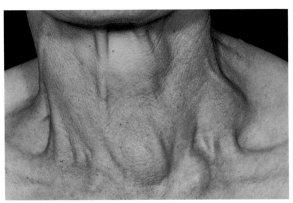

862

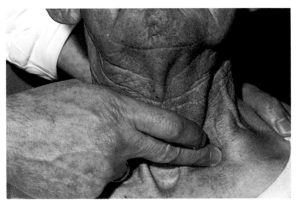

863

862–863 Signal lymph node of Virchow
More frequently than is generally appreciated the left prescalene supraclavicular lymph nodes are involved by metastatic lesions from malignant tumors in the abdomen including the urogenital tract. Dissemination takes place through the cisterna chyli. If there is reason to suspect metastases to these lymph nodes, a serial section study of the excised nodes should be performed. – Fig. **862** shows a metastasis from a colon carcinoma, and, in Fig. **863**, the primary was a prostate carcinoma. Scalene node biopsy is helpful in detecting micrometastases when there are no palpable nodes but metastases are suspected.

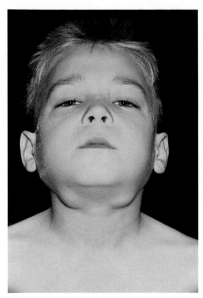

864

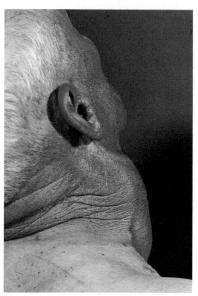

865

864 Non-Hodgkin's lymphoma, lymphoblastic lymphoma
Systemic malignant lymphoma manifested in the submandibular and parotid lymph nodes of an 8-year-old boy. Intrathoracic nodes were present. The patient died despite therapy.

865 Non-Hodgkin's lymphoma, immunoblastic sarcoma
There are large metastatic lymph nodes in the neck of this 68-year-old patient. The metastases enlarged to this size within a few weeks.

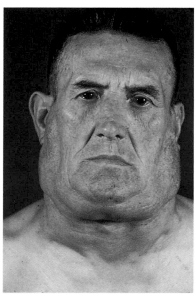

866 Chronic-lymphatic leukemia
This man had a 20-pound weight loss and swelling of the face and neck over a period of six months, and generalized adenopathy including especially the nodes of the face and the neck.

866

Index